Gluten Free Cookbook For Beginners 2024

A Fast Collection of 101+ Healthy Recipes For Busy Lifestyles

Oil-Free, Plant-Based

Nelly Berry

Disclaimer: The information provided in this cookbook is for educational and informational purposes only and is not intended as medical advice. The recipes included are based on personal experiences and preferences and may not be suitable for everyone. It is recommended to consult with a qualified healthcare professional or nutritionist before making any significant changes to your diet or lifestyle. The author and publisher disclaim any liability arising directly or indirectly from the use of the recipes or information provided in this cookbook.

Every effort has been made to ensure that the information in this book is accurate and up-to-date at the time of publication. However, the author and publisher do not assume any responsibility or liability for any errors or omissions that may occur.

Table Of Contents

Introduction To Gluten-free.

However, in today's culinary scene, being gluten-free has evolved from a simple dietary choice to one of the most important and health-conscious lifestyle choices for millions of people worldwide. For those suffering from celiac disease or gluten intolerance, the protein gluten, which is found in wheat, barley, and rye, is a major source of worry. Understanding the fundamentals of a gluten-free lifestyle and overcoming its obstacles are the main goals of this introduction.

We set out to explore the nitty-gritty of gluten and how it affects food in this quick overview. We investigate the history of gluten, examine its physiological consequences, and shed light on the health issues that require a gluten-free diet. Through a more comprehensive comprehension of gluten, readers will be able to see the significance of implementing a gluten-free diet plan for their overall health.

Choosing the right ingredients is only one aspect of maintaining a gluten-free diet. For individuals who are adopting a gluten-free lifestyle, meal planning, grocery store navigation, and eating out present particular difficulties. This book gives readers the tools they need to take charge of their nutrition and lead happy, satisfying lives without gluten by providing them with useful advice and techniques.

Let's embrace the endless opportunities that come with adopting a gluten-free lifestyle as we set out on this journey together. Whether you're following this route out of curiosity or necessity, I hope this book will be a source of inspiration and direction for you as you start your gluten-free journey. Welcome to a world where health is king and flavor has no limits. Greetings from the gluten-free world.

The Importance of Gluten-Free Living

In recent years, the importance of gluten-free living has become increasingly recognized, not only among individuals with gluten sensitivities or celiac disease but also among those seeking to optimize their health and well-being. Here, we delve into the significance of adopting a gluten-free lifestyle:

1. Managing Celiac Disease: For individuals diagnosed with celiac disease, a lifelong autoimmune disorder triggered by the ingestion of gluten, adhering to a strict gluten-free diet is paramount. Gluten consumption can lead to damage in the small intestine, resulting in a range of debilitating symptoms such as digestive issues, nutrient deficiencies, fatigue, and even long-term complications such as osteoporosis and certain cancers. By eliminating gluten from their diet, individuals with celiac disease can effectively manage their condition and prevent further harm to their health.

2. Relieves gluten sensitivity. In addition to celiac disease, many people experience non-celiac gluten sensitivity, which is characterized by adverse reactions to gluten without autoimmune markers. Symptoms can vary greatly and may include bloating, abdominal discomfort, fatigue, headaches and joint pain. Adopting a gluten-free diet may alleviate these symptoms, improving people's digestive health and overall well-being.

3. Digestive health improves. Even in people who have not been diagnosed with a gluten-related disease, consuming gluten can cause digestive discomfort and inflammation. Some people may experience a mild form of gluten intolerance, and reducing their gluten intake may improve their digestive symptoms. By adopting a gluten-free lifestyle, people can support digestive health and reduce the risk of gastrointestinal disorders.

4. Supports overall well-being. A gluten-free diet can provide a variety of health benefits beyond digestive health. For some people, going gluten-free can lead to higher energy levels, clearer skin, improved mood, and improved cognitive function. By focusing on whole, natural, gluten-free foods such as fruits, vegetables, lean proteins, and gluten-free grains, people can nourish their bodies with nutrient-dense foods that promote overall health.

5. Explore culinary diversity. Contrary to popular belief, living gluten-free does not mean deprivation or monotony. Instead, it opens up a world of culinary possibilities and encourages people to explore a diverse range of gluten-free ingredients, flavors and dishes. From ancient grains like quinoa and amaranth to gluten-free foods for baking and cooking, a gluten-free diet brings creativity and innovation to the kitchen.

UNDERSTANDING GLUTEN

What's Gluten

Gluten is a protein composite found in certain grains, primarily wheat, barley, and rye. It is responsible for the elastic texture of dough and gives bread its chewy texture. Gluten consists of two main proteins: glutenin and gliadin. While gluten is harmless for most people, it can trigger adverse reactions in individuals with celiac disease, wheat allergies, or non-celiac gluten sensitivity. For them, consuming gluten can lead to digestive issues, autoimmune reactions, and other health problems. As a result, gluten-free diets have become essential for managing these conditions and promoting overall well-being.

Effects Of Gluten On The Body

The effects of gluten on the body can vary significantly depending on individual factors such as genetics, immune response, and underlying health conditions. For most people, consuming gluten poses no harm and is a normal part of their diet. However, for individuals with certain gluten-related disorders, gluten can have profound and often adverse effects on their health. Here are some of the effects of gluten on the body:

1. Celiac Disease: In individuals with celiac disease, consuming gluten triggers an autoimmune response that damages the lining of the small intestine. This can lead to a range of symptoms, including abdominal pain, bloating, diarrhea, constipation, fatigue, weight loss, nutrient deficiencies, and in severe cases, long-term complications such as osteoporosis, infertility, and certain cancers.

2. Non-Celiac Gluten Sensitivity: Some individuals experience adverse reactions to gluten despite not having celiac disease or a wheat allergy. This condition, known as non-celiac gluten sensitivity, can manifest with symptoms such as bloating, abdominal discomfort, diarrhea, constipation, fatigue, headaches, joint pain, and skin problems. While the exact mechanism is not fully understood, avoiding gluten-containing foods typically alleviates these symptoms.

3. Wheat Allergy: Wheat allergy is an immune-mediated reaction to proteins found in wheat, including gluten. When individuals with a wheat allergy consume gluten, their immune system identifies it as a threat and produces antibodies to fight it, leading to allergic symptoms such as hives, itching, swelling, difficulty breathing, nausea, vomiting, diarrhea, and in severe cases, anaphylaxis.

4. Neurological and Psychiatric Symptoms: Some individuals with gluten-related disorders,

particularly celiac disease, may experience neurological and psychiatric symptoms due to gluten exposure. These can include headaches, migraines, brain fog, difficulty concentrating, anxiety, depression, irritability, and mood swings. In some cases, adopting a gluten-free diet can improve or alleviate these symptoms.

5. Systemic Inflammation: Gluten consumption has been implicated in promoting systemic inflammation in some individuals, even those without diagnosed gluten-related disorders. Chronic inflammation is linked to various health conditions, including cardiovascular disease, diabetes, autoimmune disorders, and neurodegenerative diseases. For some people, reducing or eliminating gluten from their diet may help reduce inflammation and improve overall health.

Conditions Requiring A Gluten-free Diet

1. Celiac Disease:

Celiac disease is an autoimmune disorder characterized by an abnormal immune response to gluten, a protein found in wheat, barley, and rye.

In individuals with celiac disease, consuming gluten triggers an immune reaction that damages the lining of the small intestine, leading to inflammation and interfering with nutrient absorption.

Symptoms of celiac disease can vary widely and may include abdominal pain, bloating, diarrhea, constipation, fatigue, weight loss, nutrient deficiencies, skin rashes, and neurological issues.

A strict gluten-free diet is the only treatment for celiac disease, as consuming gluten can exacerbate symptoms and lead to long-term complications such as malnutrition, osteoporosis, infertility, and certain cancers.

2. Non-Celiac Gluten Sensitivity:

Non-celiac gluten sensitivity refers to adverse reactions to gluten in individuals who do not have celiac disease or wheat allergy.

While the exact mechanism is not fully understood, consuming gluten can trigger symptoms such as abdominal pain, bloating, diarrhea, constipation, fatigue, headaches, joint pain, and skin problems in people with non-celiac gluten sensitivity.

Diagnosis of non-celiac gluten sensitivity is based on the exclusion of celiac disease and wheat allergy, and symptom improvement on a gluten-free diet.

3. Wheat Allergy:
Wheat allergy is an immune-mediated reaction to proteins found in wheat, including gluten.

In individuals with a wheat allergy, consuming gluten can trigger an allergic response, leading to symptoms such as hives, itching, swelling, difficulty breathing, nausea, vomiting, diarrhea, and in severe cases, anaphylaxis.

Unlike celiac disease and non-celiac gluten sensitivity, wheat allergy is diagnosed through allergy testing and may require immediate medical intervention in case of severe reactions.

4. Dermatitis Herpetiformis:

Dermatitis herpetiformis is a skin manifestation of celiac disease characterized by itchy, blistering skin rashes.

It is caused by the same abnormal immune response to gluten seen in celiac disease.

Following a strict gluten-free diet can help alleviate symptoms and prevent flare-ups of dermatitis herpetiformis.

5. Gluten Ataxia:

Gluten ataxia is a neurological condition characterized by damage to the cerebellum, resulting in symptoms such as poor coordination, tremors, difficulty walking, and speech disturbances.

It is believed to be caused by an immune reaction to gluten.

Treatment involves adhering to a gluten-free diet to prevent further neurological damage.

Individuals with celiac disease, non-celiac gluten sensitivity, wheat allergy, dermatitis herpetiformis, or gluten ataxia must follow a strict gluten-free diet to manage their symptoms, prevent complications, and promote their overall health and well-being. Consulting with a healthcare professional or registered dietitian is essential for proper diagnosis and guidance in adopting a gluten-free lifestyle.

Gluten Free Ingredients

Common Ingredients to Avoid

1. Wheat:
Wheat is one of the primary sources of gluten and is found in various forms, including wheat flour, wheat bran, wheat germ, and semolina.

Common wheat-based products to avoid include bread, pasta, cereal, baked goods, and flour-based sauces and gravies.

2. Barley:
Barley contains gluten and is often used in brewing beer, malted beverages, and certain cereal grains.

Ingredients derived from barley, such as barley malt extract, barley malt syrup, and barley malt flavoring, should be avoided.

3. Rye:
Rye is another grain that contains gluten and is commonly found in bread, crackers, cereals, and certain alcoholic beverages.

Ingredients derived from rye, such as rye flour, rye bread, and rye whiskey, should be excluded from a gluten-free diet.

4. Triticale:
Triticale is a hybrid grain derived from crossing wheat and rye, making it unsuitable for gluten-free diets.

Products containing triticale, such as some bread, cereal, and baked goods, should be avoided.

5. Durum:
Durum wheat is a variety of wheat that is often used in pasta production.

Pasta made from durum wheat contains gluten and should be replaced with gluten-free alternatives such as rice or corn pasta.

6. Semolina:
Semolina is a coarse flour made from durum wheat and is commonly used in pasta, couscous, and certain baked goods.
Due to its gluten content, semolina should be avoided on a gluten-free diet.

7. Farro:
Farro is an ancient grain related to wheat and contains gluten.
While it is considered nutritious, individuals following a gluten-free diet should opt for gluten-free grains such as quinoa, rice, or buckwheat instead.

8. Spelt:
Spelt is an ancient wheat variety that contains gluten and is commonly used in bread, pasta, and baked goods.

Despite its popularity as a health food, spelt is not suitable for individuals with gluten-related disorders.

9. Bulgur:
Bulgur is a type of wheat that has been partially cooked, dried, and cracked, making it a quick-cooking grain used in salads, pilafs, and side dishes.
Due to its gluten content, bulgur should be avoided on a gluten-free diet.

10. Hydrolyzed Wheat Protein:
Hydrolyzed wheat protein is a common ingredient in processed foods, soups, sauces, and condiments.
Despite being processed, it still contains gluten and should be avoided by individuals following a gluten-free diet.

Avoiding these common ingredients containing gluten is essential for individuals adhering to a gluten-free diet to prevent adverse reactions and promote overall health and well-being. Reading food labels carefully and choosing naturally gluten-free alternatives are crucial steps in maintaining a gluten-free lifestyle.

Gluten-Free Alternatives

1. Gluten-Free Grains:
Quinoa: A nutritious gluten-free grain rich in protein, fiber, and various vitamins and minerals. Rice (including brown rice, white rice, and wild rice): Versatile and widely available, rice serves as a staple in many gluten-free diets.

- Buckwheat: Despite its name, buckwheat is not related to wheat and is naturally gluten-free. It can be used in porridge, pancakes, and baked goods.

- Millet: A small grain with a mildly sweet flavor, millet is gluten-free and suitable for use in pilafs, porridge, and baked goods.

- Amaranth: High in protein and fiber, amaranth is a gluten-free grain that can be cooked similarly to rice or used in baking.

- Sorghum: A whole grain that is naturally gluten-free and rich in fiber and antioxidants. Sorghum flour can be used in baking.

2. Gluten-Free Flours and Starches:
Almond flour: Made from ground almonds, almond flour is a popular gluten-free alternative in baking.

- Coconut flour: Made from dried coconut meat, coconut flour is high in fiber and adds a subtle coconut flavor to baked goods.

- Tapioca flour/starch: Tapioca flour, derived from the cassava root, adds chewiness and texture to gluten-free baking.

- Arrowroot starch: A fine powder extracted from the roots of tropical plants, arrowroot starch is used as a thickening agent in gluten-free recipes.

- Potato starch: Made from the starch of potatoes, potato starch is often used in gluten-free baking to add lightness and moisture to baked goods.

3. Gluten-Free Pasta:

There are numerous gluten-free pasta options available, made from alternative grains such as rice, corn, quinoa, chickpeas, or lentils. These pasta varieties offer similar taste and texture to traditional wheat-based pasta.

4. Gluten-Free Bread and Baked Goods:

Gluten-free bread and baked goods are made using a combination of gluten-free flours, starches, and binding agents. These products are widely available in stores or can be homemade using gluten-free flour blends and recipes.

5. Whole Foods:

Many whole foods are naturally gluten-free and can serve as nutritious alternatives to gluten-containing products. Fruits, vegetables, legumes, nuts, seeds, eggs, poultry, fish, and meat are all naturally gluten-free and can form the basis of a balanced gluten-free diet.

6. Gluten-Free Oats:

While oats themselves are gluten-free, they are often contaminated with gluten during processing. Certified gluten-free oats are available for individuals with celiac disease or gluten sensitivity to enjoy oats without the risk of cross-contamination.

MANAGING THE DIET

Planning Meals

Meal planning is essential for individuals following a gluten-free diet to ensure they have access to safe and nutritious meals throughout the week. Here are some tips for effective meal planning on a gluten-free diet:

1. Create a Weekly Meal Plan:
Set aside time each week to plan your meals for the upcoming days. Consider your schedule, dietary preferences, and any special occasions or events that may impact your meals.

2. Focus on Naturally Gluten-Free Foods:
Build your meals around whole, naturally gluten-free foods such as fruits, vegetables, lean proteins, legumes, nuts, seeds, and gluten-free grains like rice, quinoa, and millet.

3. Embrace Variety:
Incorporate a diverse range of ingredients and flavors into your meals to keep things interesting and ensure you're getting a wide range of nutrients. Experiment with different cuisines, cooking techniques, and seasonal produce.

4. Batch Cook and Prep Ingredients:
Save time during the week by batch cooking and prepping ingredients in advance. Cook grains, proteins, and vegetables in large batches and store them in portioned containers for quick and easy meals throughout the week.

5. Plan for Leftovers:
Intentionally cook extra portions of meals to have leftovers for future lunches or dinners. Leftovers can be a lifesaver on busy days when you don't have time to cook from scratch.

6. Read Labels and Check Recipes:
When planning meals, carefully read labels on packaged ingredients to ensure they are gluten-free. Look for gluten-free certification or

labels, and be cautious of hidden sources of gluten.

Choose recipes from trusted sources that are explicitly labeled as gluten-free or use naturally gluten-free ingredients. Modify recipes as needed to make them gluten-free by substituting gluten-containing ingredients with gluten-free alternatives.

7. Incorporate Convenience Foods Wisely:
While whole, unprocessed foods are ideal, it's also okay to incorporate gluten-free convenience foods like pre-packaged gluten-free pasta, bread, and snacks into your meal plan occasionally. Just be sure to check labels for gluten-free certification or safe ingredients.

8. Plan for Dining Out:
If you anticipate eating out during the week, research gluten-free-friendly restaurants in advance and check their menus online. Call ahead to inquire about gluten-free options and

ask questions about cross-contamination procedures to ensure a safe dining experience.

9. Stay Organized:
Keep your meal plan, grocery list, and recipes organized in a central location such as a meal planning app, notebook, or calendar. This will help you stay on track and avoid last-minute scrambling.

Grocery Shopping Tips

Grocery shopping can be a breeze when you're following a gluten-free diet with a little preparation and knowledge. Here are some tips to help you navigate the aisles and select gluten-free options with confidence:

1. Make a List:
Before heading to the store, create a list of gluten-free foods and ingredients you need for

the week. Organize your list by categories such as fruits, vegetables, proteins, grains, dairy, and pantry staples to ensure you don't forget anything.

2. Read Labels Carefully:
When selecting packaged foods, carefully read the ingredient labels to identify any gluten-containing ingredients such as wheat, barley, rye, or their derivatives. Look for products labeled as "gluten-free" or certified gluten-free by reputable organizations.

3. Choose Naturally Gluten-Free Foods:
Focus on whole, unprocessed foods that are naturally gluten-free, such as fruits, vegetables, lean proteins, legumes, nuts, seeds, dairy, and gluten-free grains like rice, quinoa, and oats (if certified gluten-free).

4. Be Wary of Cross-Contamination:
Be cautious of cross-contamination, especially in bulk bins, deli counters, and shared equipment. Look for dedicated gluten-free sections or

products that are certified gluten-free to minimize the risk of cross-contact with gluten-containing foods.

5. Explore Gluten-Free Sections:
Many grocery stores now offer dedicated gluten-free sections or aisles stocked with gluten-free products. Take advantage of these sections to find a variety of gluten-free options, including pasta, bread, snacks, and baking ingredients.

6. Stock Up on Staples:
Keep your pantry stocked with gluten-free staples such as gluten-free flour blends, pasta, rice, quinoa, canned beans, canned tomatoes, gluten-free oats, nuts, seeds, nut butter, and gluten-free baking ingredients like baking powder and xanthan gum.

7. Plan Ahead for Special Occasions:
If you have a special occasion or event coming up, plan ahead by researching gluten-free options and specialty products you may need.

Consider visiting specialty stores or online retailers that offer a wide selection of gluten-free products.

8. Be Mindful of Hidden Gluten:
Be aware of hidden sources of gluten in products such as sauces, condiments, salad dressings, soups, marinades, and seasoning mixes. Look for gluten-free alternatives or make your own using gluten-free ingredients.

9. Use Shopping Apps and Resources:
Utilize smartphone apps, websites, and resources that provide information on gluten-free products, brands, and recipes. These tools can help you make informed choices and discover new gluten-free products.

10. Advocate for Yourself:
If you're unsure whether a product is gluten-free or have questions about cross-contamination, don't hesitate to ask a store employee or contact the manufacturer for clarification. Your health

and well-being are important, so advocate for yourself and seek out the information you need.

By following these grocery shopping tips, you can shop confidently for gluten-free foods and ingredients, enjoy a varied and nutritious diet, and maintain your gluten-free lifestyle with ease.

BREAKFAST AND BRUNCH RECIPES

Baked Eggs With Spinach, Tomatoes, Ricotta & Basil

Prep:10 mins Cook:30 mins Easy Serves 4-6

Kcal 271 Fat17g Saturates 5g Carbs 11g Sugars 11g Fiber 3g Protein 17g Salt 0.7g

Ingredients

- 1 tbsp olive oil
- 1 onion, finely chopped
- 1 garlic clove, crushed
- pinch of chili flakes
- 3 x 400g cans finely chopped tomatoes (or blitz regular canned chopped tomatoes using a food processor or hand blender)
- 3 tbsp sundried tomato pesto (ensure vegetarian, if needed)

- 200g spinach, roughly chopped
- 8 eggs
- 100g ricotta
- 40g parmesan or vegetarian alternative, finely grated
- handful of basil leaves
- crusty bread or focaccia, to serve

Method

STEP 1

Heat the oil and 2 tbsp butter in a large, shallow, flameproof casserole or frying pan over a low-medium heat and fry the onion with a pinch of salt for 10 mins until soft and translucent. Add the garlic and chili flakes, and fry for 1 min more. Tip in the tomatoes, 1 tsp sugar and pesto. Season and simmer, uncovered, for 10 mins, stirring often. Tip in the spinach and cook for another 5 mins until wilted.

STEP 2

Heat the grill too hot. Using the back of a spoon, make 8 wells in the sauce and crack the eggs one by one. Top with ricotta cheese and sprinkle with Parmesan cheese. Cover and cook for 5 minutes, then place under the hot grill for a few minutes until the egg whites set and the yolks runny. Sprinkle with basil and serve with crusty bread for dipping.

Keto Pancakes

Prep:5 mins Cook:20 mins Easy Serves 2

kcal 731, fat 61g, saturates 7g, low in carbs 7g, sugars 4g, fiber 0.3g, protein 38g, salt 1.15g.

Ingredients

4 eggs
75ml almond milk
1 tsp stevia
1 tsp baking powder
pinch of ground cinnamon
175g almond flour
½ tsp vanilla extract

Method

Step 1

Whisk eggs and almond milk in a bowl. Add stevia, baking powder, cinnamon, almond flour, and vanilla, then stir.

 Step 2

Heat a nonstick skillet over medium heat. Drop in two tablespoons of batter and cook until the edges set, about 2 to 3 minutes. Flip and cook for another 2 minutes until golden brown. Repeat with remaining dough, then top with your favorite toppings and serve in piles. It's topped with fried striped bacon, keto-friendly maple syrup, and just a few blueberries.

Herb Omelette With Fried Tomatoes

Prep:5 mins Cook:5 mins Easy Serves 2

Kcal 204 Fat 14g Saturated 4g Carbs 4g Sugars 4g Fiber 1g Protein 17g Salt 0.5g

Ingredients

1 tsp olive oil
3 tomatoes, halved
4 large eggs
1 tbsp chopped parsley
1 tbsp chopped basil

Method

Step 1
Heat the oil in a small non-stick frying pan and fry the tomatoes. Fry, cut side down, until soft and change color. Meanwhile, in a small bowl, whisk the eggs with the herbs and plenty of freshly ground black pepper.

Step 2
Remove the tomatoes from the pan and place on two serving plates. Pour the egg mixture into the pan and stir gently with a wooden spoon to move

any eggs that have settled to the bottom of the pan and allow the raw egg to flow into the spaces. When it is almost cooked, make an omelet without stirring. Cut into four pieces and serve with tomatoes.

Buckwheat Galettes

Prep:20 mins / Cook:30 mins / Easy / Serves 4

Kcal 411 Fat 25g Saturates 13g Carbs 20g Sugars 4g Fiber 1g Protein 25g Salt 1.7g

Ingredients
- 80g buckwheat flour
- 5 medium eggs
- 250ml milk
- 2 tsp Dijon mustard
- 4 tbsp single cream
- 100g mature gruyère, comté or cheddar, grated
- butter, for frying
- 100g ham, torn

- fried mushrooms or steamed spinach, to serve (optional)

Method

Step 1

In a kettle or bowl, mix the flour, 1 egg, milk and a pinch of salt. Let it sit for 30 minutes or up to 3 hours. In a separate bowl, combine mustard, cream, and cheese. Preheat the oven to 200C/180C fan/gas 6. Line two baking trays with parchment paper or foil.

Step 2

Melt the butter in a large skillet, then add enough batter to cover the pan once it bubbles and swirl to coat the surface with a thin layer (pour any remaining batter back into the batter bowl). Cook until the surface hardens and the underside turns slightly brown, then carefully turn over and cook for another 1 to 2 minutes and then turn off the heat.

Step 3

Spoon a quarter of the cheese mixture into the center of the pancake, using the spoon to make space in the center for the egg. Divide one into spaces and place a few slices of ham around the edges. Fold both sides of the pancake toward the center to form a square. Cook in the pan for another 30 seconds to 1 minute, then transfer to the baking sheet. Repeat with remaining pancakes and bake until egg whites set, 6 to 7 minutes. Serve with sautéed mushrooms or wilted spinach, if desired.

Avocado & Black Bean Eggs

Prep:5 mins /Cook:5 mins / Easy / Serves 2

Kcal 356 Fat 20g Saturates 4g Carbs 18g Sugars 5g Fiber 11g Protein 20g Salt 0.8g

Ingredients

2 tsp rapeseed oil
1 red chilli, deseeded and thinly sliced

1 large garlic clove, sliced
2 large eggs
400g can black beans
½ x 400g can cherry tomatoes
¼ tsp cumin seeds
1 small avocado, halved and sliced
handful fresh, chopped coriander
1 lime, cut into wedges

Method

STEP 1

Heat oil in a large nonstick skillet. Add the peppers and garlic and cook until soft and change color. Break an egg on both sides of the pan. Once they begin to set, arrange the beans (and their juice) and tomatoes around the pan and sprinkle with cumin seeds. The goal is to reheat the beans and tomatoes, not cook them.

STEP 2

Remove the pan from the heat and sprinkle with the avocado and coriander. Squeeze half of the lime wedges. Serve, leaving any remaining wedges to shrink on the sides.

Turkish One-Pan Eggs & Peppers (Menemen)

Prep:10 mins / Cook:25 mins / Easy / Serves 4

Kcal 222 Fat 15g Low In Saturates 4g Carbs 12g Sugars 9g fiber 3g Protein 12g Low In Salt 0.39g

Ingredients
2 tbsp olive oil
2 onions, sliced
1 red or green pepper, halved deseeded and sliced
1-2 red chillies, deseeded and sliced
400g can chopped tomatoes
1-2 tsp caster sugar
4 eggs
small bunch parsley, roughly chopped
6 tbsp thick, creamy yogurt
2 garlic cloves, crushed

Method

STEP 1

Heat oil in a heavy-bottomed frying pan. Add onion, pepper, and chili powder. Cook until it begins to soften. Add tomatoes and sugar and mix well. Cook and season until   liquid evaporates.

Step 2

Using a wooden spoon, create 4 pockets in the tomato mixture and crack in the eggs. Cover the pan and cook over low heat until the eggs set.

Step 3

Add garlic to yogurt and mix. Sprinkle the parsley over the menemen and add a dollop of garlicky yogurt to the pan.

Mushroom Brunch

Prep:5 mins / Cook:12 mins - 15 mins / Easy /
Serves 4

Kcal 154 Fat 11g Saturates 2g Carbs 1g Sugars
1g Fiber 2g Protein 13g Salt 0.4g

Ingredients

250g mushrooms
1 garlic clove
1 tbsp olive oil
160g bag kale
4 eggs

Method

STEP 1
Chop the mushrooms and crush the garlic
cloves. Heat the olive oil in a large skillet and
sauté the garlic over low heat for 1 minute. Add
mushrooms and cook until soft. Then add
cabbage. If the cabbage doesn't all fit in the pan,
add half, stir until wilted, then add the rest.

When the cabbage is completely wilted, season it.

Step 2

Now break the egg and cook it on low heat for 2-3 minutes. Then cover and wait another 2-3 minutes or until the eggs are cooked to your liking. For a keto-friendly version, serve with regular or keto bread.

Healthy Shakshuka

Prep:10 mins / Cook:30 mins / Easy / Serves 2

Kcal 342 Fat 17g Saturates 3g Carbs 21g Sugars 19g Fiber 10g Protein 21g Salt 0.5g

Ingredients

1 tbsp cold pressed rapeseed oil
1 red onion, cut into thin wedges
1 red pepper, finely sliced
1 yellow pepper, finely sliced

3 large garlic cloves, crushed
1 tsp cumin seeds
1 tsp coriander seeds, crushed
1 heaped tsp sweet smoked paprika
400g can cherry tomatoes
115g baby spinach
4 medium eggs
½ small bunch coriander, roughly chopped
½ small bunch dill, roughly chopped

Method

STEP 1
Heat oil in a large nonstick skillet. Add the onions and peppers and cook over medium heat until the vegetables are soft, 8 to 10 minutes. Add garlic, cumin, coriander and paprika and cook for 1 minute more. Add tomatoes, spinach, and 100ml of water and boil until the spinach wilts. Then, reduce the heat, cover, and simmer for 10 minutes. Season to taste.

Step 2

Make four holes in the tomato mixture and carefully crack an egg into each hole. Cover with a lid or foil and cook over low heat for 8 to 10 minutes or until the eggs are set. Open the lid, sprinkle with fresh herbs and enjoy..

LUNCH RECIPE

Broccoli And Kale Green Soup

Prep:15 mins Cook:20 mins Easy Serves 2

kcal 182 low in fat 8g saturates 1g carbs 14g sugars 4g fiber 5g protein 10g salt 0.7g

Ingredients

- 500ml stock, made by mixing 1 tbsp bouillon powder and boiling water in a jug
- 1 tbsp sunflower oil
- 2 garlic cloves, sliced
- thumb-sized piece ginger, sliced
- ½ tsp ground coriander
- 3cm/1in piece fresh turmeric root, peeled and grated, or 1/2 tsp ground turmeric
- pinch of pink Himalayan salt
- 200g courgettes, roughly sliced
- 85g broccoli
- 100g kale, chopped

- 1 lime, zested and juiced
- small pack parsley, roughly chopped, reserving a few whole leaves to serve

Method

STEP 1

Heat oil in a deep frying pan, add garlic, ginger, coriander, turmeric, and salt and fry over medium heat for 2 minutes. Add 3 tablespoons of water to slightly moisten the seasoning.

Step 2

Add the courgettes, toss well to coat the slices with all the spices, and continue cooking for another 3 minutes. Add 400ml of broth and boil for 3 minutes.

Step 3

Add broccoli, kale, and lime juice to the remaining broth. Cook again for 3 to 4 minutes until all vegetables are tender.

Step 4

Turn off the heat and add the chopped parsley. Pour everything into a blender and blend on high speed until smooth. It will be a beautiful green with dark specks (i.e. cabbage). Garnish with lime zest and parsley.

Gluten-Free Sundried Tomato Bread

Prep:15 / mins Cook:1 hr / Easy / Makes 1 loaf

A quick, gluten-free bread recipe - no need for yeast, ready in under an hour

kcal 74 fat 3g saturates 1g carbs 10g sugars 0g fiber 1g protein 3g low in salt 0.7g

Ingredients

- 200g gluten-free white flour
- 1 tsp salt
- 3 tsp gluten-free baking powder
- 284ml buttermilk (or same amount of whole milk with a squeeze of lemon juice)

- 3 eggs
- 1 tsp tomato purée
- 2 tbsp olive oil
- 50g sundried tomatoes in oil (about 6-8), coarsely chopped
- 25g parmesan (or vegetarian parmazano), grated

Method

STEP 1

Preheat the oven to 180°C/fan 160°C/gas. 4. Combine flour, salt, and baking powder in a large bowl. In a separate bowl, mix together the buttermilk, eggs, tomato puree, and oil. Mix the wet and dry ingredients, then add the sun-dried tomatoes and half the Parmesan cheese.

Step 2

Grease a 900g loaf pan and pour the mixture into it. Sprinkle the remaining Parmesan cheese on top and bake for 50 to 60 minutes until a skewer inserted in the center comes out clean. Transfer to a wire rack to cool.

Minty Carrot, Pistachio & Feta Salad

Prep:20 mins / Cook:30 mins Plus chilling / Easy / Serves 6

Kcal 307 Fat 20 G Saturates 6g Carbs 20g Sugar 10g Fiber 6g Protein 12g Salt 1.6g

Ingredients

- 2 tbsp olive oil, plus a little extra for drizzling
- 500g carrot, halved and cut into chunks
- 400g can chickpea, drained and rinsed
- 2 tsp ground cumin
- juice ½ lemon
- 1 tbsp clear honey
- small bunch mint, chopped
- 2 big handfuls spinach
- 100g bag shelled pistachio, roughly chopped
- 200g pack feta cheese, crumbled

Method

STEP 1
Preheat the oven to 200C/180C fan/gas. 6. Add 1 tablespoon of oil, carrots, chickpeas, and cumin to a baking sheet, season and toss. Roast for 30 minutes or until carrots are tender.

Step 2
Mix the lemon juice, honey and remaining oil and pour over the roasted carrots and chickpeas. Let it cool. At this point, the salad can be refrigerated for up to 1 day. Remove from the refrigerator 1 hour before serving.

Step 3
Mix mint, spinach leaves, and pistachios and check the seasoning. Top with feta cheese and drizzle with a little oil.

Easy Egg Muffins

Prep:15 mins / Cook:25 mins / Easy / Makes 8 (serves 4)

Kcal 229 Fat 16g Saturates 5g Carbs 2g Sugars 2g Fiber 2g Protein 17g Salt 0.6g

Ingredients

- 1 tbsp oil
- 150g broccoli, finely chopped
- 1 red pepper, finely chopped
- 2 spring onions, sliced
- 6 large eggs
- 1 tbsp milk
- large pinch of smoked paprika
- 50g cheddar or gruyère, grated
- small handful of chives, chopped (optional)

Method

STEP 1
Preheat the oven to 200C/180C fan/gas. 4. Grease an 8-hole muffin tin with half of the

butter. Add the remaining oil to the frying pan and add the broccoli, peppers, and green onions. Stir-fry for 5 minutes. Set aside to cool.

Step 2

In a bowl, whisk together the eggs, milk, smoked paprika, and half the cheese. Add cooked vegetables. Pour the egg mixture into the muffin cavities and top with the remaining cheese and a few onions, if desired. Bake for 15 to 17 minutes, or until golden brown and cooked through.

Sweet Potato, Spinach & Feta Tortilla

Prep: 5 mins / Cook: 20 mins / Easy 3 (or 2 adults and 2 children

Kcal 572 Fat 25g Saturates 9g Carbs 59g Sugars 31g Fiber 10g Protein 23g Salt 1.6g

Ingredients
- 3 sweet potatoes

- 2 tbsp olive oil
- 100g baby spinach
- 6 large eggs
- 100g feta, crumbled

Method

STEP 1

Pierce each side of the potato several times. Microwave for 5-8 minutes until soft and let cool slightly.

Step 2

Heat the oil in a 20cm ovenproof frying pan and fry the spinach for 1-2 minutes (you may need to do this in batches). Cut the potatoes in half lengthwise, scoop out the flesh with a spoon and store it in large chunks. Beat the eggs.

Step 3

Add the sweet potatoes to the pan and toss with the spinach. Don't mix too much. Pour in the eggs and stir until all the crevices in the pan are filled. Add the feta cheese and cook over low heat until lightly browned on the bottom and sides, 4 to 5 minutes.

Step 4

Place under the broiler for 1 to 2 minutes to brown the top. Check if it is cooked by piercing the center with a knife. Let cool before cutting into wedges. Refrigerate for up to 1 day.

Butternut Soup With Crispy Sage & Apple Croutons

Prep:20 mins / Cook:30 mins / Easy / Serves 4

Kcal 231 Low In Fat 7g Saturates 1g Carbs 31g Sugars 20g Fiber 8g Protein 4g Salt 0.4g

Ingredients
- 1 tbsp olive oil
- 1 large onion, chopped
- 1 garlic clove, chopped
- 1 butternut squash, about 1kg, peeled, deseeded and chopped

- 3 tbsp madeira or dry Sherry
- 500ml gluten-free vegetable stock, plus a little extra if necessary
- 1 tsp chopped sage, plus 20 small leaves, cleaned and dried
- sunflower oil, for frying
- For the apple croutons
- 1 tbsp olive oil
- 1 large eating apple, peeled, cored and diced
- a few pinches of golden caster sugar

Method

STEP 1

Heat oil in a large frying pan, add onion and fry for 5 minutes. Add garlic and pumpkin and cook for 5 more minutes. Pour in the Madeira and stock, add the chopped sage, cover and simmer for 20 minutes until the squash is tender.

Step 2

Blend with a hand blender or food processor until smooth. Let cool in the pan and refrigerate until ready to serve. Store for 2 days or freeze for up to 3 months. To make crispy sage, heat a little oil (about 2cm deep) in a small saucepan and then dip the sage leaves in it until crispy. You will need to do this in multiple steps. Drain on kitchen paper. Lasts for several hours.

Step 3

Warm the soup in a pot just before serving. The texture is quite thick and soft. If it is too thick, add a little broth to thin it out.

Step 4

For the apple croutons: Heat the oil in a large skillet, add the apples and cook until soft. Sprinkle it with sugar and stir until lightly caramelized.

Step 5

To serve, pour soup into small bowls and top with apples, sage and cracked pepper.

Easy Quinoa Salad

Prep:30 mins Cook:30 mins Easy Serves 4

kcal 404 fat 21.4g saturates 8.4g carbs 35.3g sugars 11.2g fiber 2.6g protein 17.3g salt 1.9g

Ingredients

- 200g quinoa
- 3 tbsp olive oil
- 1 red onion, peeled but left whole, then cut into 1cm thick round slices
- 2 peppers, red, yellow or mixture, deseeded and cut into chunky long wedges
- 200g baby courgette, halved lengthways
- 3 garlic cloves, unpeeled
- zest and juice 1 lemon
- pinch of sugar
- small pack flat-leaf parsley, roughly chopped
- 200g pack feta cheese

Method

STEP 1

Cook quinoa according to package directions,
then drain well and set aside.

Step 2

Meanwhile, heat the oven to 200C/180C fan/gas.
6. Add 1 tablespoon of oil and seasoning to the
onions and peppers, fry them on a baking sheet,
and bake for 15 minutes.

Step 3

Mix the pumpkin and garlic with the rest of the
vegetables and bake for another 15 minutes.

Step 4

Squeeze out the skin of the roasted garlic and
mash it with the seasoning. Add the remaining
butter, lemon juice and zest and season with
sugar. Pour over the quinoa and toss with the
roasted vegetables and parsley. Sprinkle over the
feta cheese, toss lightly again and serve.

Salsa Verde Baked Eggs

Prep:5 mins Cook:15 mins Easy Serves 4

low in kcal 268 fat 21g saturates 4g carbs 7g sugars 6g fiber 3g protein 12g salt 0.7g

Ingredients

- 5 tbsp olive oil
- 1 tsp smoked paprika
- 1 tsp cumin seeds
- 400g can cherry tomatoes
- 200g fresh cherry tomatoes
- 2 garlic cloves
- 1 small bunch of parsley
- 1 small bunch of basil
- ½ small bunch of mint, leaves picked
- 2 tbsp capers
- 1 tsp Dijon mustard
- 2 tbsp white wine vinegar
- 200g baby spinach, washed
- 4 eggs
- ½ tsp chili flakes (optional)
- flatbreads, to serve (optional)

Method

STEP 1

Add 1 tablespoon of olive oil to a frying pan or frying pan and fry the paprika and cumin over medium heat for 30 seconds. Add canned and fresh tomatoes, bring to a boil, cover, and simmer over medium heat until tomatoes are soft, 5 to 6 minutes.

Step 2

Meanwhile, blend garlic, most of the parsley, basil, mint, capers, mustard, white wine vinegar, 4 tablespoons oil, and 3 tablespoons cold water in a food processor until a smooth paste forms. season.

Step 3

Add the spinach to the pan with the tomatoes and stir until wilted (cover again for a few minutes and stir again until wilted). Dip into the mixture four times and carefully crack the eggs. Cover and cook over medium heat for 6 to 8 minutes or until eggs are fully cooked. Open the pan lid and pour the herb sauce. Sprinkle with remaining parsley and chili flakes, if using. Serve with flatbread, if desired.

Tuna, Avocado & Quinoa Salad

Prep:5 mins Cook:20 mins Easy Serves 2

kcal 663 fat 44g saturates 10g carbs 34g sugars 7g fiber 8g protein 28g salt 1.1g

Ingredients
- 100g quinoa
- 3 tbsp extra virgin olive oil
- juice 1 lemon
- ½ tbsp white wine vinegar
- 120g can tuna, drained
- 1 avocado, stoned, peeled and cut into chunks
- 200g cherry tomatoes on the vine, halved
- 50g feta, crumbled
- 50g baby spinach
- 2 tbsp mixed seeds, toasted

Method

STEP 1
Rinse the quinoa in cold water. Put it in a pot, add water and boil. Reduce the heat and simmer for 15 minutes, until the grains are puffed but still have some flavor. After draining the water, transfer to a bowl and cool slightly.

Step 2
Meanwhile, in a kettle, combine the oil, lemon juice and vinegar with some seasoning.

Step 3
Once the quinoa has cooled, add the dressing and all other ingredients and mix. Please put it on a plate or lunch box.

Mackerel & Potato Salad With Lemon Caraway Dressing

Prep:10 mins Cook:15 mins Easy Serves 2

kcal 558 fat 43g saturates 8g carbs 20g sugar 8g
fiber 4g protein 23g salt 2.1g

Ingredients

- 175g small new potato
- 200g smoked mackerel fillets, skin removed
- 4 spring onions, finely sliced
- 140g small cooked beetroot, sliced into wedges
- small bunch dill, finely chopped
- 2 tbsp olive oil
- juice 1 lemon, zest of half
- ¼ tsp caraway seeds

Method

STEP 1

Place the potatoes in a small saucepan of boiling water and simmer for 15 mins or until fork-tender. Cool and cut into thick slices.

STEP 2

Flake the mackerel into a bowl and add the cooled potatoes, spring onions, beetroot and dill.

STEP 3

In a separate bowl, whisk together the olive oil, lemon juice, caraway seeds and some seasoning. Pour over the salad and toss everything well to coat. Scatter over the lemon zest. Pack into plastic containers and chill, or eat straight away.

DINNER RECIPES

Paneer Korma

Prep:5 mins / Cook:25 mins / Easy / Serves 4

Kcal 509 Fat 29 Gsaturates 12g Carbs 21g Sugars 12g Fiber 16g Protein 33g salt 0.7g

Ingredients

- 3 tbsp vegetable oil
- 225g block of paneer, cut into 2cm cubes
- 1 large onion, roughly chopped
- thumb-sized piece of ginger, peeled
- 2 large garlic cloves
- 5 tbsp korma paste
- 3 cardamom pods, crushed
- 70g ground almonds
- 500ml vegetable stock
- 150g spinach
- 100g Greek yogurt
- rice or naan breads, to serve (optional)

Method

STEP 1

Heat 1 tablespoon of oil in a deep skillet over medium heat. Add the paneer cubes and fry for 5 minutes, turning regularly, until golden brown on each side. Take it out with tongs and place it on a plate lined with kitchen paper.

Step 2

Place the onion, ginger, and garlic in a food processor, add a little water, and pulse until smooth. Heat remaining oil in a skillet over medium heat. Add the onion mixture and a pinch of salt and sauté for 10 minutes or until lightly golden. Add korma paste and cardamom and fry for 1 minute. Add almond powder and stir-fry for 1 minute to make a thick batter.

Step 3

Add broth, bring to a boil, and simmer, uncovered, for 5 to 10 minutes or until slightly reduced. Add spinach to the sauce and cook for

5 minutes. Add yogurt and paneer and season generously. Eat with rice or warm naan bread.

Prawn Tikka Masala

Prep:10 mins / Cook:30 mins / Easy / Serves 4

Kcal 432 Fat 16g Saturates 3g Carbs 50g Sugars 12g Fiber 5g Protein 18g Salt 1.1g

Ingredients

- 1 large onion, roughly chopped
- 1 thumb-sized piece ginger, peeled and grated
- 2 large garlic cloves
- 1 tbsp rapeseed oil
- 2-3 tbsp tikka curry paste
- 400g can chopped tomatoes
- 2 tbsp tomato purée
- ½ tbsp light brown soft sugar
- 3 cardamom pods, bashed
- 200g brown basmati rice
- 3 tbsp ground almonds

- 300g raw king prawns
- 1 tbsp double cream
- ½ bunch of coriander, roughly chopped
- naan breads, warmed, to serve (optional)

Method

Step 1

The onion, ginger, and garlic in a food processor and process until smooth. Heat oil in a large ovenproof pot or skillet over medium heat. Add the onion paste and cook for 8 minutes or until lightly golden. Add curry paste and cook for 1 more minute. Add the tomatoes, tomato puree, sugar and cardamom pods. Bring to a boil, cover and simmer for another 10 minutes.

Step 2

Prepare rice according to package directions.

Step 3

Remove the cardamom from the curry sauce, discard, and puree with a hand blender or clean food processor. Return to pan, add almonds and shrimp and cook for 5 minutes. Season to taste and add cream and cilantro. Served with rice and naan bread if desired.

Spicy Fish Stew

Prep:10 mins / Cook:40 mins / Easy
/ Serves 4

Kcal 664 Fat 26g Saturates 5g Carbs 58g Sugars 14 Fiber 14g Protein 42g Salt 0.3g

Ingredients
- 1 tbsp olive oil
- 2 onions, thinly sliced
- 3 spring onions, chopped
- 3 garlic cloves, chopped
- 1 red chilli, seeded and thinly sliced
- few thyme sprigs
- 2 x 400g cans chopped tomatoes
- 400ml vegetable bouillon made with 2 tsp vegetable bouillon powder

- 2 green peppers, seeded and cut into pieces
- 160g brown basmati rice
- 400g can and 210g can red kidney beans, drained
- handful fresh coriander, chopped, plus a few sprigs extra
- handful flat-leaf parsley, chopped
- 550g pack frozen wild salmon, skinned and cut into large pieces
- 1 lime, zested

Method

STEP 1

Heat the oil in a large nonstick skillet and fry the onion for 8 to 10 minutes until soft and golden. Add green onions, garlic, pepper, and thyme. Cook and stir for 1 minute. Pour in the tomatoes and broth and add the pepper. Cover and simmer for 15 minutes.

Step 2

Meanwhile, cook rice according to package directions. Add the beans along with the cilantro and parsley, then simmer for another 10 minutes until the peppers are tender. Add salmon and lime zest and cook until tender, 4 to 5 minutes.

Step 3
Pour into a bowl and sprinkle with coriander.

Peanut Butter Chicken

Prep:10 mins / Cook:40 mins / Easy / Serves 4

Kcal 572 Fat 43g Saturates 20g Carbs 11g Sugars 7g Fiber 3g Protein 33g Salt 0.3g

Ingredients
- 2tbsp avocado oil
- 8 skinless boneless chicken thighs, cut into chunks
- 1 onion, finely chopped
- 3 garlic cloves, crushed

- 2 red chillies, finely sliced (deseeded if you don't like it too hot)
- 2tsp fresh ginger, grated
- 2tbsp garam masala
- 100g smooth peanut butter
- 400ml coconut milk
- 400g can chopped tomatoes
- coriander, ½ roughly chopped, ½ leaves picked
- roasted peanuts, to serve
- cauliflower rice to serve

Method

STEP 1

Heat 1 tablespoon of oil in a deep skillet over medium heat. Fry the chicken in batches until golden brown and set aside. Sauté for 8 minutes until the onions are soft. Then stir in the remaining 1 tablespoon garlic, pepper and ginger. L. Add 1 minute of oil and garam masala and cook for another minute.

Step 2

Add peanut butter, coconut milk, and tomatoes and bring to a boil. Return the chicken to the pan and add the chopped cilantro. Simmer for 30 minutes until the sauce has thickened and the chicken is cooked through.

Step 3
Serve with remaining coriander, roasted peanuts and rice, if desired.

Creamy Garlic, Lemon & Spinach Salmon

Prep:5 mins / Cook:15 mins / Easy / Serves 2

Kcal 721 Fat 44g Saturates 16g Carbs 34g Sugars 19g Fiber 7g Protein 43g Salt 0.5g

Ingredients
- 2 sweet potatoes
- 1 tbsp olive oil or rapeseed oil
- 2 salmon fillets, skin removed
- 2 garlic cloves, thinly sliced

- 170g baby spinach
- 1 lemon, zested and ½ juiced, ½ thinly sliced
- 75g mascarpone
- 5 tbsp milk

Method

STEP 1

Preheat the oven to 200C/180C fan/gas. 6. Prick each sweet potato a few times and microwave for 5 minutes until tender (or bake for 35 to 40 minutes). Keep warm until serving.

Step 2

Pour half of the oil into a frying pan and lightly sear the salmon on both sides. Don't worry about it overcooking at this stage. Transfer the salmon to a plate, wipe out the pan, and heat the remaining oil. Cook for 30 seconds, making sure the garlic doesn't brown, then add the spinach, lemon zest, juice, and a few seasonings. Add mascarpone and 2 tablespoons milk and cook until spinach is wilted.

Step 3

 Place the spinach mixture in an ovenproof dish and top with the lemon slices and salmon filets. Grill for 5-8 minutes until salmon is cooked through.

Step 4

 Meanwhile, peel the sweet potato and mash it with the remaining milk and seasoning. Serve sweet potato puree with salmon and creamed spinach.

Fennel-Roasted Cauliflower With Quinoa

Prep:15 mins / Cook:40 mins / Easy / Serves 4
Healthy
Vegetarian

Kcal 260 Fat 10g Saturates 2g Carbs 27g Sugars 14g Fiber 9g Protein 10g Salt 0.1g

Ingredients

- 1 large cauliflower, or 2 small ones, separated into florets
- 1 tbsp fennel seeds
- 1 tsp coriander seeds
- 1 tsp smoked paprika
- 2 tbsp olive oil
- 1 red onion, chopped
- 2 peppers (mix of red, yellow or orange), chopped
- 1 courgette, halved lengthways, cored and chopped
- 1 small garlic clove, crushed
- 1 lemon, juiced and zested
- 4 tbsp yogurt
- 250g quinoa, cooked

Method

STEP 1

Preheat the oven to 200C/180C fan/gas. 6. Boil salted water in a large pot and boil the cauliflower for 5 minutes. Drain and place on a surface to allow excess water to evaporate.

Step 2

Crush the fennel and coriander seeds with a pestle and mortar, then mix with the paprika and some seasoning. Place the cauliflower in a large bowl, drizzle with half the olive oil and sprinkle with the spice mixture. Toss the florets until completely coated.

Step 3

Place the inflorescences on a baking sheet, arranging them at a distance from each other. Place the red onions, peppers and zucchini on a separate baking sheet, drizzle with the remaining oil and cook for 30 to 35 minutes. Cook until browned on all sides and slightly crispy in parts.

Step 4

Mix the garlic with lemon juice and add the yogurt. If necessary, add a little water to thicken. Toss the roasted onions, peppers and zucchini with the cooked quinoa, lemon zest and a pinch of salt.

Step 5

Place the quinoa salad on a plate and top with the cauliflower florets. Sprinkle it with garlic yogurt.

Gluten-Free Salmon Pasta

Prep:10 mins / Cook:5 mins / Easy / Serves 2

Kcal 587 Fat 15g Saturates 7g Carbs
86g Sugars 3g Fiber 6g Protein 24g Salt 2.1g

Ingredients

- 1 gluten-free vegetable stock cube
- 200g gluten-free pasta, such as penne or fusilli
- 100g green beans, trimmed
- 100g smoked salmon, roughly chopped
- 50g baby spinach
- 1 spring onion, finely sliced
- 50g soft cheese (ensure it's gluten-free)
- ½-1 lemon, juiced
- 1 tbsp grated parmesan

Method

STEP 1

Bring a large pot of salted water to a boil, then add the stock cubes and stir to dissolve. Add pasta and cook according to package directions, about 8 to 10 minutes. Add the mung beans 1 minute before the end of cooking.

Step 2

Drain the pasta and green beans, reserving some of the cooking water. Return the pasta and beans to the pan and add the smoked salmon, spinach, green onions, and soft cheese. Add a little pasta water to soften the cheese into a sauce, then season with salt and freshly ground pepper. Squeeze lemon juice to taste and mix well. Serve with Parmesan cheese.

Black Pepper Chicken & Lemon Yogurt

Prep:45 mins / Cook:30 mins plus 1 hr marinating / Easy / Serves 4

Kcal 486 Fat 35g Saturates 13g Carbs 7g Sugars 5g Fiber 1g Protein 34g Salt 1.1g

Ingredients

- 1 tbsp black peppercorns
- 5 garlic cloves, grated, plus 1 whole garlic bulb
- 1 tsp ground turmeric
- 2 lemons, 1 juiced, plus extra wedges to serve
- 1 ½ kg whole chicken, spatchcocked (see tip, below)
- 1 tbsp olive oil
- 400g Greek yogurt
- small bunch of coriander, roughly chopped (optional)
- peppered rice, to serve (see 'goes well with')

Method

STEP 1

Crush the peppercorns using a pestle and mortar. Add minced garlic and ½ teaspoon salt and blend until a thick paste forms. Add turmeric and lemon juice and set aside.

Step 2

Place the chicken on a plate, skin side up, cutting evenly over the entire surface. Rub the marinade all over the chicken until completely coated, then cover and refrigerate for at least 1 hour, preferably overnight.

Step 3

Preheat the oven to 220C/200C fan/gas. Place the chicken, skin side up, on a shallow baking sheet and place the garlic bulbs next to it. Drizzle most of the chicken and some garlic with oil. Roast for 30 minutes, then remove the garlic bulbs from the pan and set aside. Continue roasting the chicken for another 10 to 15 minutes, or until the chicken is crispy and cooked through. If you have a food thermometer, it should read at least 65°C when inserted into the breast and at least 70°C when inserted into the thigh. Place the chicken on the baking sheet and let sit, uncovered, for 10 to 15 minutes.

Step 4
Meanwhile, peel and squeeze the garlic from the fried onions into a bowl, then stir into the yogurt. After the chicken has rested, lift it out onto the board and add the pan juices to the yogurt. Taste the yogurt and add a little more lemon juice if needed. Cut the chicken into pieces and serve, if desired, topped with yogurt sauce, peppery yellow rice (recipe below), lemon wedges and a sprinkling of coriander.

Iraqi Lamb Kofta Kebabs

Prep:25 mins / Cook:1 hr / Easy / Serves 4 - 6

Kcal 327 Fat 26g Saturates 11g Carbs 4g Sugars 3g Fiber 4g Protein 17g Salt 1.3g

Ingredients

- 3 garlic cloves, crushed or grated
- thumb-sized piece of ginger, peeled and finely grated
- 2 shallots, roughly chopped
- small handful of parsley, roughly chopped
- 2 mint sprigs, leaves picked and roughly chopped
- 2 tsp ground cumin
- 2 tsp ground coriander
- 1 tsp ground cinnamon
- 1 tbsp tomato purée
- 500g lamb mince
- 1 tbsp chopped coriander
- 2 tbsp pomegranate seeds
- hummus, fattoush salad, flatbreads and tzatziki, to serve (optional)
- For the aubergines
- 6 baby aubergines
- 4 tbsp olive oil
- 2 tsp ground cumin
- 75g butter
- 2 tbsp harissa

Method

STEP 1

Let's deal with the branches first. Preheat the oven to 180C/160C fan/gas. 4. Cut the eggplant in half lengthwise, then make a cross-shaped incision, being careful not to go all the inside. Combine oil and cumin in a small bowl and mix well. Brush the eggplants with this. Bake for 45 minutes or until tender. Remove to a platter.

Step 2

Melt the butter in a small skillet and fry the harissa for a few minutes with a pinch of salt. Pour this over the cooked eggplant.

Step 3

Meanwhile, place garlic, ginger, shallot, parsley, mint half, cumin, coriander, cinnamon, tomato purée, 1 teaspoon each salt, and freshly ground pepper in the food processor. Pulse until everything is finely chopped, about 30 seconds.

Step 4

 Place lamb in a large bowl and add seasoning mixture, stirring until well combined. If using bamboo skewers, soak them for 15 minutes before continuing.

Step 5

 Form the lamb mixture into meatballs and place on skewers. Roll the meat with your hands until it forms an egg shape. Continue until all mixture has been used.

Step 6

 Heat the grill to high heat and sear the kofta for about 6 minutes, then flip and cook for another 6 minutes until the meat is cooked through. Place the koftas on top of the eggplants and sprinkle with the remaining mint, coriander and pomegranate seeds. Serve with hummus, fattoush salad, flatbreads or tzatziki, if desired.

Puy Lentil Salad With Beetroot & Walnuts

Prep:5 mins / No cook / Easy / Serves 2

Kcal 495 Fat 27g Saturates 3g Carbs 38g Sugars 19g Fiber 15g Protein 18g Salt 0.6g

Ingredients

- ½ the lentil base from the puy lentils with salmon (recipe below)
- 2 cooked beetroots (160g), halved and sliced
- 8 walnut halves, roughly chopped
- 4 tbsp mint, roughly chopped
- 2 handfuls of rocket
- balsamic vinegar, for drizzling

Method

STEP 1
Spoon half of the remaining lentil base from the baked salmon recipe into two bowls or lunch containers and top with beets, walnuts, mint and arugula.

Step 2

Just before serving, sprinkle with balsamic vinegar and stir.

GLUTEN-FREE SNACK RECIPES

Gluten-Free Lemon Drizzle Cake

Freezable (without drizzle) Gluten-free Nut-free

Kcal 514 Fat 36g Saturates 2g Carbs 41g Sugars 35g Fiber 2g Protein 9g Salt 0.88g

Ingredients
- 200g butter, softened
- 200g golden caster sugar
- 4 eggs
- 175g ground almond (switch for polenta or wheat-free flour to make this recipe nut-free)
- 250g mashed potato
- zest 3 lemons
- 2 tsp gluten-free baking powder
- For the drizzle
- 4 tbsp granulated sugar

- juice 1 lemon

Method

STEP 1
Preheat the oven to 180C/fan 160C/gas. 4. Grease and line a 20cm deep round cake tin. Beat the sugar and butter until light and fluffy, then gradually add the eggs, beating after each addition. Add almonds, cold mashed potatoes, lemon zest, and baking powder.

Step 2
Place in the pan, level the top, and bake for 40-45 minutes, or until a skewer inserted in the center comes out golden brown. Let cool for 10 minutes, then transfer to a wire rack. Mix the granulated sugar and lemon juice, then spoon it onto the top of the cake and let it drip down the sides. Let the cake cool completely before cutting.

Gluten-Free Carrot Cake

Freezable (Freeze uniced) Gluten-free

Nutrition: per serving
Kcal 599 Fat 28g Saturates 16g Carbs 86g
Sugars 64g Fiber 2g Protein 6g Salt 0.6g

Ingredients

- 140g unsalted butter, softened, plus extra for greasing
- 200g caster sugar
- 250g carrots, grated
- 140g sultanas
- 2 eggs, lightly beaten
- 200g gluten-free self-raising flour
- 1 tsp cinnamon
- 1 tsp gluten-free baking powder
- 50g mixed nut, chopped
- For the icing
- 75g butter, softened
- 175g icing sugar
- 3 tsp cinnamon, plus extra for dusting

Method

STEP 1

Preheat the oven to 180C/160C fan/gas. 4. Grease   a 900g/2lb loaf tin and line with parchment paper.

Step 2

Cream the butter and sugar until creamy, then add the grated carrots and raisins. Add eggs to the mixture little by little.

Step 3

Add the flour, cinnamon, baking powder and most of the chopped nuts and mix well. Spoon the mixture into the loaf pan and bake for 50-55 minutes, or until a skewer inserted in the center comes out clean. Let cool in the pan for 15 minutes, then remove from the pan and cool completely on a wire rack.

Step 4

Meanwhile, make the glaze. In a large bowl, beat the butter until very soft, then add the brown sugar and cinnamon, then beat until thick and creamy. Once the cake has cooled, spread the frosting on top, sprinkle with a little more cinnamon and sprinkle with the remaining chopped nuts.

Spicy Chickpeas

Prep:5 mins / Cook:25 mins / Easy / Serves 4

Carbs 10g Sugars 0g Fiber 3g Protein 4.5g Salt 0.41g

Ingredients

- 400g can chickpea, drained and dried
- 1 tsp vegetable oil
- 1 tbsp chilli powder
- Our Most Popular Alternative
- Spicy chickpea stew

Method

STEP 1

Place the chickpeas in a bowl with the vegetable oil and chili powder and toss until the chickpeas are coated with the chili. Transfer to a baking sheet, spread the chickpeas and cook for 25 minutes. Take it out of the oven and let it cool. Sprinkle it with sea salt before serving.

Apple Crisps

Prep:5 mins / Cook:40 mins / Easy Makes roughly 16

Kcal 5 Fat 0g Saturates 0g Carbs 1g Sugars 1g Fiber 0g Protein 0g Salt 0.1g

Ingredients

1 apple

Method

STEP 1

Preheat the oven to 140C/120C fan/gas. 1. Cut apples into thin slices through the core. To get thin slices, use a mandoline if you have one. Place slices on a parchment-lined baking sheet and bake for 40 minutes. Cool until crispy.

Energy Balls With Dates

Prep:10 mins / No cook / Easy / Makes 6

Nutrition: per serving
Kcal 113 Fat 3g Saturates 1g Carbs 21g Sugars 18g Fiber 2g Protein 2g Salt 0g

Ingredients
- 50g soft dried apricot
- 100g soft dried date
- 50g dried cherry
- 2 tsp coconut oil
- 1 tbsp toasted sesame seed

Method

STEP 1
Place the apricots, dates, and cherries in a food processor and pulse until very finely chopped. Place in a bowl and apply coconut oil with your hands. Form the mixture into walnut-sized balls, then roll in sesame seeds. Store in an airtight container until you need a quick energy boost.

Dukkah-Crusted Squash Wedges

Prep:15 mins / Cook:30 mins / Easy / Serves 4

Kcal 282 Fat 14g Saturates 1g Carbs 28g Sugars 15g Fiber 9g Protein 7g Salt 0.1g

Ingredients
- 50g blanched hazelnuts
- 1 tbsp coriander seeds
- 2 tbsp sesame seeds
- 1 tbsp ground cumin
- 1 large butternut squash

- 1 tbsp olive oil

Method

STEP 1

Preheat the oven to 200C/180C fan/gas. 6. Add the hazelnuts to the skillet and fry over medium heat until golden brown. Add the coriander and sesame seeds and fry for 1 minute. Set aside, let cool, then add cumin powder and mash with a pestle and mortar.

Step 2

Peel the pumpkin, remove the seeds and cut into pieces. Mix the wedges with the butter, then add the dukkah coating. Place in a single layer on a baking sheet and bake for 30 to 40 minutes, rotating halfway through, until cooked through.

GLUTEN-FREE APPETIZERS

Roasted Shrimp Cocktail With Lemon-Horseradish Aioli

YIELDS: 6 serving(s)
PREP TIME: 10 mins
TOTAL TIME: 20 mins
CAL/SERV: 246

Calories 246 Fat 17 g Saturated fat
3 g Trans fat 0 g Cholesterol 190 mg Sodium
326 mg Fiber 0 g Sugar 0 g Protein 23

Ingredients

- 1/2 c. mayonnaise
- 2 tbsp. prepared horseradish
- 1/4 tsp. finely grated lemon zest, plus 2 tsp. fresh lemon juice
- 1 1/2 lb. medium shrimp, peeled, deveined
- 2 tsp. extra-virgin olive oil
- Kosher salt
- Freshly ground black pepper
- 1 tsp. chopped fresh parsley

Method

Step 1

In a small bowl, combine mayonnaise, horseradish, and lemon juice. Refrigerate until set, about 30 minutes.

Step 2

Preheat the oven to 400°. Pat shrimp dry with paper towels and place in a medium bowl. Add oil; Season with salt and pepper and mix.

Step 3

Place shrimp 1/2 inch apart on foil-lined baking sheets. Cook, turning halfway through, until pink and cooked through, 5 to 6 minutes.

Step 4

Transfer shrimp to a plate. Store at room temperature or refrigerated. Top aioli with lemon zest and parsley; Season with pepper and serve together.

Cranberry Whipped Feta Dip

6 - 8 serving(s) / PREP TIME: 10 mins / TOTAL TIME: 25 mins / CAL/SERV: 290

Ingredients

- 1/3 c. fresh orange juice, plus 1 tsp. finely grated orange zest
- 2 tbsp. honey, divided
- 1 c. fresh or frozen cranberries
- 1 sprig thyme, plus 2 tsp. chopped thyme leaves
- 6 oz. feta in brine, cut into small cubes
- 1 clove garlic, grated or minced
- 1/4 tsp. crushed red pepper flakes
- 6 oz. cream cheese, room temperature
- 2 tbsp. extra-virgin olive oil
- 2 tbsp. toasted chopped pistachios
- Crackers or crostini, for serving

Directions

Step 1

Heat a small saucepan over medium heat, mix orange juice and 1 tablespoon honey until smooth, then bring to a boil. Add cranberries and thyme sprigs and return to a boil. Reduce the heat to medium-low and cook, stirring occasionally, until the cranberries burst and taste fragrant, 7 to 8 minutes. Remove the thyme and add the orange zest. Cool down.

Step 2

Meanwhile, drain the brine from the feta. In a food processor, pulse the feta cheese, garlic, red pepper flakes, and chopped thyme until the feta cheese is finely chopped. Add cream cheese and beat until smooth. With the engine running, add the oil and stir until the mixture is smooth and fluffy.

Step 3

Transfer the whipped feta cheese to a serving bowl. Top with cooled cranberry sauce. Sprinkle with pistachios and drizzle with remaining 1 tablespoon honey. Serve with crackers.

Step 4

Prepare in advance: The dive can be completed up to 4 days in advance. Store in an airtight container and refrigerate.

Baked Salmon Sushi Cups

YIELDS: 12 / PREP TIME: 15 mins / TOTAL TIME: 40 mins

Ingredients
- Cooking spray
- 2 c. cooked sushi rice
- 3 nori sheets, quartered
- 1 (1 1/2-lb.) skinless salmon fillet, cut into 1/2" cubes
- 2 scallions, thinly sliced, plus more for serving
- 1 tsp. toasted sesame oil
- 4 tbsp. Japanese mayonnaise (such as Kewpie), divided
- 2 1/4 tsp. sriracha, divided
- Kosher salt

- 2 tsp. black and white sesame seeds

Directions

Step 1

Place a rack in the upper third of the oven. Preheat to 400°. Lightly coat a standard 12-cup muffin pan with cooking spray. Place 1 tablespoon of sushi rice in the center of each seaweed piece. Place the seaweed in the prepared pan, rice side up. Using a spoon, carefully spoon the rice into an even layer on the bottom of the cup.

Step 2

In a large bowl, mix salmon, chives, oil, 2 tablespoons mayonnaise, 2 teaspoons sriracha, and 1/4 teaspoon salt until smooth. Divide salmon mixture among muffin cups (about 1/4 cup each) and top with rice.

Step 3

Cook until salmon is almost cooked through, about 11 minutes.

Step 4

Turn on the grill and cook, being careful not to burn the salmon, until the top is charred and the salmon is cooked through, 2 to 4 minutes. Let cool for 5 minutes.

Step 5

Meanwhile, in a small bowl, combine remaining 2 tablespoons mayonnaise and 1/4 teaspoon sriracha.

Step 6

Place the sushi cup on a plate. Sprinkle with mayonnaise mixture. Sprinkle it with sesame seeds and green onions.

Reuben Pickle Bites

YIELDS: 4 - 6 Serving(s) / Prep Time: 15 Mins / Total Time: 25 mins

Ingredients

FOR THE DRESSING
  - 2 tbsp. mayonnaise
  - 2 tbsp. low-sugar ketchup
  - 1 tbsp. sweet pickle relish
  - 3/4 tsp. prepared horseradish
  - 1/2 tsp. fresh lemon juice
  - 1/4 tsp. Worcestershire sauce
  - Kosher salt
  - Freshly ground black pepper

FOR THE BITES
  - 2 c. pickle chips, drained
  - 4 oz. thinly sliced corned beef
  - 3 oz. thinly sliced Swiss
  - 1/4 c. sauerkraut

Directions

Step 1
Prepare dressing: In a small bowl, combine mayonnaise, ketchup, pickles, horseradish, lemon juice, and Worcestershire sauce. Season with salt and pepper.

Step 2

Place half of the pickle chips on a plate. Top with chopped corned beef, Swiss cabbage and sauerkraut and drizzle with dressing. Cover bites with the remaining half of the pickle and a toothpick.

Bacon-Wrapped Scallops

YIELDS: 4 serving(s) / Prep Time: 10 Mins / Total Time: 30 Mins / CAL/SERV: 356

Ingredients
- 1 lb. dry sea scallops (about 14)
- Kosher salt
- Freshly ground black pepper
- 8 oz. bacon (about 7 strips, not thick-cut)
- 2 tbsp. unsalted butter
- 1 clove garlic, smashed
- 1 tbsp. fresh thyme leaves
- Lemon wedges, for serving

Directions

Step 1

Preheat the oven to 425°. Line a rimmed baking sheet with foil.

Step 2

Pat the scallops dry with paper towels. Season with 1/2 teaspoon salt and 1/4 teaspoon pepper. Cut the bacon slices in half crosswise to create 3- to 4-inch-long strips. Wrap the bacon around the scallops and secure with toothpicks. Place scallops on a prepared sheet.

Step 3

Melt the butter in a small skillet over medium heat. Add the garlic and thyme leaves and cook, stirring, until fragrant, about 1 minute. Sprinkle the butter and thyme over the scallops, reserving the garlic in the pan.

Step 4

Grill the scallops for 15 to 20 minutes, until the bacon is crispy and the scallops are cooked through.

Step 5

 Remove the toothpick. Transfer the scallops to a plate and serve warm with lemon wedges.

Cranberry Brie Jalapeño Poppers

Yields: 2 Dz. / Prep Time: 15 Mins / Total Time: 40 mins

Ingredients

- (8-oz.) brie wheel, chopped into small pieces
- 1 1/2 c. shredded mozzarella
- 1 clove garlic, minced
- Kosher salt
- Freshly ground black pepper
- 1 (14-oz.) can whole cranberry sauce
- 12 jalapeños
- prosciutto, halved lengthwise

Directions

Step 1

Preheat oven to 400°. In a large bowl, combine brie, mozzarella cheese, and garlic. Season with salt and pepper. Add ½ can of cranberry sauce and stir to combine.

Step 2

Cut the jalapenos in half lengthwise, then remove the seeds and stems with a small spoon. Fill with cheese mixture and wrap each with half of the prosciutto.

Step 3

Place on a baking sheet and bake until the prosciutto is crisp and the peppers are tender, about 25 minutes. Serve warm with remaining cranberry sauce.

VEGAN AND VEGETARIAN RECIPES

Gluten-free Vegan recipes

Lentil Ragu With Courgetti

Prep:15 mins / Cook:40 mins / Easy / Serves 4 - 6

Kcal 578 Fat 7g Saturates 1g Carbs 87g Sugars 19g Fiber 14g Protein 35g Salt 0.2g

Ingredients
- 2 tbsp rapeseed oil, plus 1 tsp
- 3 celery sticks, chopped
- 2 carrots, chopped
- 4 garlic cloves, chopped
- 2 onions, finely chopped
- 140g button mushrooms from a 280g pack, quartered
- 500g pack dried red lentils

- 500g pack passata
- 1l reduced-salt vegetable bouillon (we used Marigold)
- 1 tsp dried oregano
- 2 tbsp balsamic vinegar
- 1-2 large courgettes, cut into noodles with a spiraliser, julienne peeler or knife

Method

STEP 1

Heat 2 tablespoons oil in a large skillet. Add the celery, carrots, garlic, and onion and cook over high heat until softened and changing color, 4 to 5 minutes. Add mushrooms and cook for 2 more minutes.

Step 2

Add lentils, passata, broth, oregano, and balsamic vinegar. Cover the pot and simmer for 30 minutes until the lentils are tender and the meat is tender. Check and stir occasionally to ensure the mixture does not stick to the bottom of the pan. If so, add a drop of water.

Step 3

Before serving, heat the remaining oil in a separate skillet, add the pumpkin and lightly fry, stirring, until soft. Serve half of the squash stew and refrigerate the rest to eat another day. Can be frozen for up to 3 months.

Tomato & Chickpea Curry

Prep:10 mins / Cook:45 mins / Easy / Serves 4

Kcal 369 Fat 23g Saturates 16g Carbs 28g Sugars 11g Fiber 6g Protein 9g Salt 0.5g

Ingredients
- 1 tbsp olive oil
- 2 onions, finely sliced
- 2 garlic cloves, crushed
- 1 tsp garam masala
- 1 tsp turmeric
- 1 tsp ground coriander

- 400g can plum tomatoes
- 400ml can coconut milk
- 400g can chickpeas, drained and rinsed
- 2 large tomatoes, quartered
- ½ small pack coriander, roughly chopped
- cooked basmati rice, to serve

Method

STEP 1
Heat 1 tablespoon of olive oil in a large frying pan and add 2 finely chopped onions. Cook until tender, about 10 minutes.

Step 2
Stir in 2 cloves of minced garlic, 1 teaspoon garam masala, 1 teaspoon turmeric, and 1 teaspoon coriander powder. Boil for 1-2 minutes, then add 400g can of plum tomatoes, mash with a wooden spoon, and boil for 10 minutes.

Step 3

Pour in a 400ml can of coconut milk and season. Bring to a boil and cook for another 10 to 15 minutes until the sauce thickens.

Step 4

Heat the chickpeas and 2 large, quartered tomatoes in a 400-gram jar that has been drained and washed. Sprinkle coarsely chopped cilantro from ½ small packet and serve with fluffy rice.

Mango Salad With Avocado And Black Beans

Cook:15 mins / No cook / Easy / Serves 2

Kcal 341 Fat 15g Saturates 3g Carbs 33g Sugars 18g Fiber 15g Protein 11g Salt 0.7g

Ingredients
- Kcal 341 Fat 15g Saturates 3g Carbs 33g Sugars 18g Fiber 15g Protein 11g Salt 0.7g
- beans, drained and rinsed

Method

STEP 1
In a bowl, combine lime zest and juice, mango, avocado, tomato, chilli and onion, then add coriander and beans.

Sweet Potato & Peanut Curry

Prep:15 mins / Cook:45 mins / Easy / Serves 4

Kcal 387 Fat 25g Saturates 18g Carbs 32g Sugars 15g Fiber 7g Protein 6g Salt 0.6g

Ingredients
- 1 tbsp coconut oil
- 1 onion, chopped
- 2 garlic cloves, grated
- thumb-sized piece ginger, grated
- 3 tbsp Thai red curry paste (check the label to make sure it's vegetarian/ vegan)
- 1 tbsp smooth peanut butter

- 500g sweet potato, peeled and cut into chunks
- 400ml can coconut milk
- 200g bag spinach
- 1 lime, juiced
- cooked rice, to serve (optional)
- dry roasted peanuts, to serve (optional)

Method

STEP 1

Melt 1 tablespoon of coconut oil in a saucepan over medium heat and soften 1 finely chopped onion for 5 minutes. Add 2 cloves of minced garlic and a thumb-sized piece of grated ginger and cook for 1 minute, until fragrant.

Step 2

Add 3 tablespoons of Thai red curry paste, 1 tablespoon of peanut butter, 500g of sweet potato, peel and finely chop, then add 400ml of coconut milk and 200ml of water.

Step 3

Bring to a boil, reduce heat, and simmer, uncovered, for 25 to 30 minutes or until sweet potatoes are tender.

Step 4
Add 200g of spinach and the juice of 1 lime and mix well. Serve with rice and sprinkle with a few dried roasted nuts if you want some crunch.

Easy Vegan Chocolate Cake

Prep:30 mins / Cook:25 mins plus cooling / Easy / Serves 12 - 16

Kcal 452 Fat 24g Saturates 6g Carbs 53g Sugars 34g Fiber 3g Protein 4g Salt 0.9g

Ingredients

For the cake
- a little dairy-free sunflower spread, for greasing

- 1 large ripe avocado (about 150g)
- 300g light muscovado sugar
- 350g gluten-free plain flour
- 50g good-quality cocoa powder
- 1 tsp bicarbonate of soda
- 2 tsp gluten-free baking powder
- 400ml unsweetened soya milk
- 150ml vegetable oil
- 2 tsp vanilla extract

For the frosting

- 85g ripe avocado flesh, mashed
- 85g dairy-free sunflower spread
- 200g dairy-free chocolate, 70% cocoa, broken into chunks
- 25g cocoa powder
- 125ml unsweetened soya milk
- 200g icing sugar, sifted
- 1 tsp vanilla extract
- gluten-free and vegan sprinkles, to decorate

Method

STEP 1

Preheat the oven to 160C/140C fan/gas. 3. Spread a little dairy-free sunflower paste on two 20cm sandwich tins and line the bottom with baking parchment.

Step 2

Place 1 large avocado and 300g light muscovado sugar in a food processor and pulse until smooth.

Step 3

Add 350g gluten-free flour, 50g cocoa powder, 1 tsp. Soda, 2 teaspoons. Gluten-free baking powder, 400ml unsweetened soy milk, 150ml vegetable oil and 2 tsp. ½ tsp vanilla extract. Add good salt and stir again. On a velvety dough.

Step 4

Divide the batter among the pans and bake for 25 minutes, or until the cake is fully risen and a skewer inserted in the center comes out clean.

Step 5

 Let cool in the pan for 5 minutes, then invert the cake onto a wire rack to cool completely.

Step 6

 While you wait, start making the frosting. Beat 85g ripe avocado flesh and 85g dairy-free sunflower paste with an electric beater until creamy and smooth. Pass through a sieve and set aside.

Step 7

 Melt 200g of dairy-free chocolate in a bowl of water or in the microwave, then leave to cool for a few minutes.

Step 8

 Sift 25g cocoa powder into a large bowl. Boil 125ml of unsweetened soy milk and add to the cocoa, gradually stirring until smooth. Let cool for a few minutes.

Step 9

Add the avocado mixture, 200g sifted brown sugar, melted chocolate and 1 teaspoon vanilla, stirring constantly to form a shiny, thick glaze. Use this to make sandwiches and top cakes.

Step 10

Top with sprinkles or desired decorations and let sit for 10 minutes before slicing. Available up to 2 days in advance.

GLUTEN-FREE VEGETARIAN RECIPES

Vegetarian Thai Green Curry

Prep:15 mins / Cook:40 mins / Easy / Serves 4

Kcal 339 Fat 26g Saturates 15g Carbs 17g Sugars 11g Fiber 7g Protein 6g Salt 0.6g

Ingredients
- 2 tbsp vegetable oil
- 3 shallots, finely sliced
- 4 tbsp Thai green curry paste

- 1 red chili, deseeded and finely chopped
- 350g butternut squash, peeled and cut into 1.5cm cubes
- 1 large red pepper, deseeded and cut into thick slices
- 400g can full fat coconut milk
- 5 lime leaves
- 150g mangetout
- 100g baby corn. halved lengthways
- 1 small bunch coriander, roughly chopped
- cooked rice and lime wedges, to serve

Method

STEP 1

Heat the oil in a large ovenproof pot with a tight-fitting lid. Add the shallots, season generously with salt and cook over medium heat until soft and beginning to caramelize, 7 to 10 minutes. Add the curry paste and chili peppers to the plate and fry for 2 minutes. Add pumpkin and pepper, followed by 200ml coconut milk and water. Add the lime leaves, cover, and simmer for 15 to 20 minutes, or until the squash is tender.

STEP 2

Stir the mangetout and baby corn through the curry, then re-cover, cooking over a medium-low heat for a further 5 mins or until the veg is just cooked. Season and stir through half the coriander. Remove the lime leaves and discard. Spoon the curry into deep bowls, scatter with the remaining coriander and serve with rice and lime wedges for squeezing over.

Asparagus & New Potato Frittata

Prep:10 mins / Cook:12 mins / Easy / Serves 3

Kcal 310 Fat 18g Saturates 6g Carbs 16g Sugars 6g Fiber 4g Protein 19g Salt 0.7g

Ingredients
- 200g new potatoes, quartered
- 100g asparagus tips

- 1 tbsp olive oil
- 1 onion, finely chopped
- 6 eggs, beaten
- 40g cheddar, grated
- rocket or mixed leaves, to serve

Method

STEP 1

Heat the grill to high. Place potatoes in a pot of cold salted water and bring to a boil. Bring to a boil and cook for 4 to 5 minutes until almost tender, then add the asparagus and cook for another minute. drain water

Step 2

Meanwhile, heat oil in an oven-safe frying pan and add onion. Cook until tender, about 8 minutes.

Step 3

Add the eggs and half the cheese to the container and mix well. Add the onions to the pan and scatter over the asparagus and potatoes.

Sprinkle the remaining cheese on top and place under the grill for 5 minutes, or until golden brown and cooked through. Cut into pieces and serve with salad.

Aubergine, Halloumi & Harissa Skillet Bake

Prep:10 mins / Cook:40 mins / Easy / Serves 2

Kcal 546 Fat 39g Saturates 20g Carbs 15g Sugars 14g Fiber 7g Protein 31g Salt 3.5g

Ingredients
- 2-4 tbsp olive oil, plus a drizzle
- 1 large aubergine, sliced into rounds about ½cm thick
- 2 large garlic cloves, crushed
- 400g can chopped tomatoes
- 1 tbsp harissa paste
- ½ tsp caster sugar
- 225g block halloumi, sliced into 8-9 pieces

- pinch of dried mint
- flatbreads, rice or couscous, to serve

Method

STEP 1

Heat 1 tablespoon of the oil in an ovenproof frying pan or frying pan about 8 inches (22 cm) in diameter, then add the eggplant slices in a single layer (you will need to do this in batches). Cook 2 to 3 minutes on each side until golden and tender, adding 1 tablespoon more oil between each serving. Transfer to a plate.

Step 2

If the pan is dry, add 1 tablespoon more. L. Saute until the emulsified garlic begins to sizzle but does not change color. Add the tomatoes, harissa, sugar, and a pinch of salt. Mash the tomatoes and bubble for 1 minute. Turn off the heat and let cool slightly.

Step 3

Meanwhile, cut the halloumi pieces in half (don't worry if they fall apart). Arrange the eggplant and halloumi slices in overlapping concentric circles on top of the tomato mixture, making sure there is a slice or two of halloumi between each eggplant slice. Drizzle with a little more oil and sprinkle with mint. Cover the tin with foil and bake at 180C/160C fan/gas 4 for 20 minutes. Then remove the foil and bake for another 5-10 minutes until the halloumi is browned. Serve with warm flatbreads, rice or couscous.

Halloumi Traybake

Prep:15 mins / Cook:1 hr / Easy / Serves 4

Kcal 564 Fat 24g Saturates 8g Carbs 53g Sugars 15g Fiber 12g Protein 28g Salt 1.6g

Ingredients
- 750g baby new potatoes, halved

- 2 medium red onions, quartered and broken up into large pieces
- 4 tbsp olive oil
- 400g can chickpeas, drained
- 1 large red pepper, sliced into strips
- ½ romanesco broccoli or cauliflower (about 400g), cut into small florets
- 250g mixed colour cherry tomatoes
- 4 garlic cloves, peeled
- 250g pack reduced fat halloumi, thinly sliced
- small bunch basil, leaves torn

Method

STEP 1

Preheat the oven to 160°C/140°C fan/gas. 3. Place potatoes with onions in a large baking dish. Add 2 tablespoons of olive oil and bake in the oven for about 30 minutes.

Step 2

Add chickpeas, peppers, romanesco, tomatoes, and garlic. Drizzle with 2 tablespoons of oil and bake for another 20 to 25 minutes until cooked through and browned. Stir slightly and top with halloumi pieces. Place under the grill for 5-10 minutes or until the cheese is melted and browned (watch carefully). To serve, sprinkle with basil leaves.

Kidney Bean Curry

Prep:5 mins / Cook:30 mins / Easy / Serves 2

Kcal 282 Fat 8g Saturates 1g Carbs 33g Sugars 13g Fiber 14g Protein 13g Salt 0.1g

Ingredients

- 1 tbsp vegetable oil
- 1 onion, finely chopped
- 2 garlic cloves, finely chopped
- thumb-sized piece of ginger, peeled and finely chopped
- 1 small pack coriander, stalks finely chopped, leaves roughly shredded
- 1 tsp ground cumin

- 1 tsp ground paprika
- 2 tsp garam masala
- 400g can chopped tomatoes
- 400g can kidney beans, in water
- cooked basmati rice, to serve

Method

STEP 1

Heat oil in a large skillet over low to medium heat. Add the onion and a pinch of salt and cook over low heat, stirring occasionally, until soft and changing color. Add the garlic, ginger and cilantro stems and cook for another 2 minutes until fragrant.

Step 2

 Add the spices to the pan and cook for another minute. Everything should smell fragrant. Add finely chopped tomatoes and beans to water and bring to a boil.

Step 3

Reduce the heat and simmer for 15 minutes until the curry is nice and thick. Season to taste and serve with basmati rice and coriander leaves.

GLUTEN-FREE DESSERTS RECIPES

Refreshing Lychee & Lime Sorbet

Prep:15 mins Plus freezing Easy Serves 6

kcal 137 fat 0g saturates 0g carbs 35g sugars 35g fiber 1g protein 16g salt 0.04g

Ingredients

- 3 x cans lychees in syrup
- 50g caster sugar
- egg white
- zest from 2 limes, juice from 1

Method

STEP 1

Pour two cans of lychee syrup into a small saucepan. Add sugar and melt over low heat. Boil for 1 minute.

Step 2

Place dried lychees in a food processor and pulse until very finely chopped. Pour in the lime juice and syrup, continuing to swirl the blade. Don't worry if the mixture isn't perfectly smooth at this point. Pour into a 1-liter container and freeze for at least 6 hours until firm.

Step 3

Mash the frozen mixture and return to the processor bowl. Add the egg whites and beat until thick, pale, and smooth. Add the zest of 1 lime. Put it back in the container and freeze again. Ideally, do this overnight. Scoop out the remaining lychee peel by the spoonful and sprinkle it on top.

Chocolate, Cardamom & Hazelnut Torte

Prep:30 mins Cook:40 mins Easy Serves 8

kcal 473 fat 37g saturates 15g carbs 24g sugars 21g fiber 4g protein 10g salt 0.4g

Ingredients
- 150g blanched hazelnuts
- 8 green cardamom pods
- 150g gluten-free dark chocolate
- 125g butter
- 6 eggs, separated
- 125g golden caster sugar
- 1 tbsp cocoa powder, plus extra for dusting
- crème fraîche, to serve

Method

STEP 1

Toast the hazelnuts in a dry frying pan until golden brown, then cool slightly and pulse in a food processor until finely ground. Remove the cardamom seeds from the pod and grind them using a pestle and mortar.

Step 2

Preheat the oven to 160C/140C fan/gas. 3. Butter the bottom of a 23cm springform pan and melt the chocolate and butter in the microwave for 30 seconds at a time until shiny and smooth. Let cool slightly.

Step 3

In a very clean bowl, using an electric beater, beat the egg whites until stiff peaks form. Then, without scraping the whisk, beat the yolks and sugar in a separate bowl until pale and plump.

Step 4

Mix the chocolate with the egg yolk mixture, then add the cocoa powder, a pinch of salt, cardamom seeds and hazelnuts. Stir a tablespoon of egg white into the batter to loosen the mixture, then fold in the rest to retain as much air as possible. Gently pour into the tin and bake for 35 mins. Leave to cool in the tin, then dust with cocoa powder and serve with crème fraîche.

Chocolate Orange Tart

Prep:15 mins plus soaking and chilling. No cook
Easy Serves 12

kcal 391 fat 29g saturates 19g carbs 23g sugars
20g fiber 7g protein 7g salt 0g

Ingredients
- For the filling
- 75g dates
- zest 2 oranges, juice of 1
- 50g coconut oil
- 175g clear honey
- 140g raw cacao powder (find it in health food shops or online), plus extra for dusting
- For the crust
- 100g coconut oil
- 140g ground almonds
- 175g desiccated coconut
- 2 ½ tbsp clear honey
- 1 tbsp raw cacao powder

Method

STEP 1

Place the jujubes in a bowl, pour boiling water over them, and let sit for 20 minutes. Meanwhile, pulse the crust ingredients in the food processor until smooth. Place the mixture into a loose-bottomed 23cm pie tin, using your fingers to spread it evenly across the bottom and press into the fluted sides. Cover with plastic wrap and refrigerate while you prepare the filling.

Step 2

Drain the dates and place them in a blender along with the zest and juice of 1 orange, coconut oil, honey and cocoa. Blend until smooth, then scrape off the cooled crust and smooth it out with the back of a spoon. Refrigerate for at least 1 hour. 10 minutes before serving, remove from the refrigerator and sprinkle with remaining orange zest and additional cocoa.

Gluten-Free Brownies

Prep:20 mins Cook:40 mins Easy Serves 12

kcal 515 fat 33g saturates 19g carbs 45g sugars
37g fiber 4g protein 7g salt 0.34g

Ingredients
- 250g unsalted butter, cubed, plus extra for the tin
- 250g dark chocolate, roughly chopped
- 4 large eggs
- 300g golden caster sugar
- ½ tsp vanilla extract or paste
- 100g gluten-free plain flour, sieved
- 60g cocoa powder
- ½ tsp fine sea salt
- 150g milk chocolate, roughly cut into chunks

Method

STEP 1

Preheat the oven to 180C/160C fan/gas. 4. Grease a 30cm x 20cm non-stick mold and line the bottom with non-stick baking paper.

Step 2

 Fill a small pot about 1/3 full with water, bring it to a boil and place a heatproof bowl that fits tightly on top. Add the butter and chocolate and gently melt over low heat, stirring occasionally. Be careful not to let it stick and burn to the bottom. Turn off the heat and let cool slightly.

Step 3

 Beat eggs and sugar with an electric beater for 8 to 10 minutes, or until thick enough to hold traces. Carefully add the cooled melted chocolate and vanilla, followed by the flour, cocoa and salt. Lastly, fold in the chocolate pieces. Pour the brownie batter into the pan, place in the center of the oven and bake for 30-35 minutes.

Step 4

Let cool slightly in the pan before cutting into 12 squares.

Gluten-free Apple Crumble

Prep:10 mins Cook:35 mins - 40 mins Easy Serves 4 - 6

kcal 357 fat 15g saturates 9g carbs 52g sugars 28g fiber 2g protein 3g salt 0.33g

Ingredients
- 600g Bramley apples, cut into 2cm dice
- 1 tsp ground mixed spice or cinnamon
- 2 tbsp caster sugar
- cream or vanilla ice cream, to serve
- For the crumble topping
- 100g butter, diced
- 150g gluten-free plain flour
- 75g light muscovado sugar
- 3 tbsp gluten-free porridge oats

Method

STEP 1
Preheat the oven to 190C/170C fan/gas. 5. Place apples, spices, and powdered sugar in a pot and add 2 tablespoons of water. Cover and cook gently for 5 minutes until the apples are soft, then transfer to an ovenproof dish.

Step 2
Meanwhile, rub the butter into the flour, then add the light muscovado sugar, rolled oats and a pinch of salt. Sprinkle mixture evenly over apples.

Step 3
Place the pan on a baking sheet and bake for 35-40 minutes, until the top is golden and the apples are tender. Let cool for 5 minutes and serve with cream, ice cream or custard.

Date, Banana & Rum Loaf Cake

Prep:15 mins Cook:1 hr More effort Cuts into 10 slices

kcal 310 fat 8g saturates 1g carbs 57g sugars 49g fiber 3g protein 5g salt 0.39g

Ingredients
- 250g pack stoned, ready-to-eat dates
- 2 small or 1 large banana (140g/5oz in weight)
- 100g pecans, 85g/3oz roughly chopped, rest left whole
- 200g raisins
- 200g sultanas
- 100g fine polenta
- 2 tsp mixed spice
- 2 tsp baking powder (use gluten-free if needed)
- 3 tbsp dark rum
- 2 egg whites
- a few banana chips and 1 tsp sugar (optional), to decorate

Method

STEP 1

Preheat the oven to 180°C/fan, 160°C/gas. 4. Line a 900g loaf tin with non-stick baking paper and apply a little oil to help it stick. Put the jujubes in a small pot, add 200ml boiling water, and boil for 5 minutes. Pour the liquid into a container and place the dates in a food processor. Add the banana and 100ml date liquid and whisk until smooth. Mix the nuts, dried fruit, polenta, spices and baking powder in a bowl, then add the date puree and rum and stir until smooth.

Step 2

Beat egg whites until soft peaks and add to cake mixture. Spoon into the pan (it will be quite full) and top with the remaining pecans, banana chips, and sugar (if using). Bake for 1 hour, until the pastry is golden brown and crisp and a skewer comes out clean. Let cool completely before cutting into pieces.

Raspberry Brûlée

Prep:15 mins Cook:30 mins plus 4 hrs chilling
Easy Serves 4

kcal 523 fat 46g saturates 27g carbs 22g sugars
22g fiber 1g protein 5g salt 0.1g

Ingredients
- 1 vanilla pod
- ½ lemon, pared zest only
- 300ml double cream
- 100g raspberries
- 4 egg yolks
- 2 tbsp golden caster sugar
- 2 tbsp demerara sugar

Method

STEP 1
Split the vanilla bean, scrape out the seeds, and
add to the pot with the lemon zest and cream.
Throw in a pod too. Heat the cream until it

boils and small bubbles begin to form at the edges. Turn off the heat and leave for 15 minutes.

Step 2

Preheat the oven to 160C/140C fan/gas 3. Place 4 ramekins in a baking dish and fill the tins with boiling water until the ramekins open about 2 cm.

Step 3

Divide the raspberries among the molds, reserving a few. Beat egg yolks and powdered sugar with an electric beater until very pale and fluffy, about 3 minutes. Remove the zest and vanilla bean from the cooled cream and slowly fold into the egg mixture. Transfer to a container, pour through a sieve into ramekins, then top with remaining raspberries. Bake in the oven for 20 to 25 minutes, until the custard forms a crust and shakes slightly when pushed in the pan. Let cool and refrigerate for at least 4 hours.

Step 4

If you don't have a torch, heat the grill too high. Sprinkle demerara sugar over each ramekin and use a blowtorch to caramelize the top, or place under the broiler until the sugar melts and becomes crispy. Let sit for 5 minutes before serving.

Butterscotch Pudding

Prep:20 mins Cook:10 mins plus at least 4 hrs chilling Easy Serves 4 - 6

kcal 499 fat 39g saturates 24g carbs 31g sugars 25g fiber 0g protein 5g salt 0.3g

Ingredients
- 2½ tbsp cornflour
- 3 egg yolks (freeze the whites for another recipe)
- 500ml whole milk
- 300ml double cream
- 50g butter

- 125g light muscovado sugar
- grated dark chocolate, to serve (optional)

Method

STEP 1
Whisk cornmeal and egg yolks in a bowl or pitcher. Pour half the milk and cream into a second container and set aside.

Step 2
 Melt the butter in a large saucepan with the sugar over low heat until the sugar has dissolved, about 2 to 3 minutes. Increase heat to medium and cook until caramelized, 1 to 2 minutes, being careful not to burn the sugar. Remove from heat and gradually whisk in cream mixture. Do this slowly and carefully, as the hot sugar mixture may spread slightly.

Step 3
 Return to the heat and bring to a boil, stirring constantly. Turn off the heat and add 3-5 tablespoons of the egg yolk/cornmeal mixture to

thin it out slightly, then pour it all into the pan and stir. Stir again over medium heat until the mixture boils and thickens into a custard. Remove from heat, pour into 4 to 6 glasses or ramekins and refrigerate until set, 4 hours or overnight.

Step 4

Just before serving, whip the remaining 150ml of cream with an electric whisk and pour over the pudding. Grind the chocolate if you wish.

MEAT AND SEAFOOD GLUTEN-FREE RECIPES

Grilled Lemon Herb Chicken:

Prep Time: 10 mins
Marinating Time: 30 mins
Cook Time: 15 mins
Total Time: 55 minutes
Servings: 4
Calories per serving: 250 calories

Ingredients:
- 4 boneless, skinless chicken breasts
- 2 tablespoons olive oil
- 2 cloves garlic, minced
- 1 teaspoon dried thyme
- 1 teaspoon dried rosemary
- Zest and juice of 1 lemon
- Salt and pepper to taste

Method:

Step 1.
In a bowl, whisk together olive oil, minced garlic, thyme, rosemary, lemon zest, and lemon juice.

Step 2.
Season chicken breasts with salt and pepper, then coat with the marinade. Let marinate in the refrigerator for at least 30 minutes.

Step 3.
Preheat the grill to medium-high heat. Grill chicken breasts for 6-8 minutes per side, or until cooked through and juices run clear.

Step 4.
Serve grilled lemon herb chicken with your favorite gluten-free side dishes, such as roasted vegetables or quinoa salad.

Baked Lemon Garlic Salmon:

Prep Time: 10 mins / Cook Time: 12-15 mins
Total Time: 25 minutes / Servings: 4
Calories per serving: 300 calories

Ingredients:
- 4 salmon filets
- 2 tablespoons olive oil
- 2 cloves garlic, minced
- Zest and juice of 1 lemon
- 1 teaspoon dried oregano
- Salt and pepper to taste

Method

Step 1.
 Preheat the oven to 375° F (190°c). baking line using parchment paper.

Step 2.

In a small bowl, mix together the olive oil, minced garlic, lemon zest, lemon juice, dried oregano, salt, and pepper.

Step 3.

Place salmon filets on a prepared baking sheet. brush the tops of the filets with the lemon-garlic mixture.

Step 4.

Bake in the preheated oven for 12 to 15 minutes, or until the salmon is cooked through and easily pulled apart with a fork.

Step 5.

serve grilled lemon garlic salmon with steamed vegetables and rice or gluten-free pasta.

Shrimp Stir-Fry with Vegetables:

Prep Time: 15 minutes / Cook Time: 10 minutes
Total Time: 25 minutes / Servings: 4
Calories per serving: 200 calories

Ingredients:

- 1 lb (450g) large shrimp, peeled and deveined
- 2 tablespoons gluten-free soy sauce or tamari
- 1 tablespoon sesame oil
- 2 cloves garlic, minced
- 1 teaspoon grated ginger
- 2 cups mixed vegetables (such as bell peppers, broccoli, carrots, and snap peas)
- Cooked rice or rice noodles for serving
- Instructions:

Step 1

In a bowl, toss shrimp with gluten-free soy sauce or tamari, sesame oil, minced garlic, and grated ginger. Let marinate for 15-20 minutes.

Step 2.

Heat a large skillet or wok over medium-high heat. Add marinated shrimp and cook for 2-3 minutes, or until pink and cooked through. Remove shrimp from skillet and set aside.

Step 3.

In the same skillet, add mixed vegetables and stir-fry for 3-4 minutes, or until crisp-tender.

Step 4.

Return cooked shrimp to the skillet and toss with the vegetables until heated through.

Step 5.

Serve shrimp stir-fry with cooked rice or rice noodles.

Grilled Honey Garlic Shrimp Skewers:

Prep Time: 20 mins / Marinating Time: 30 mins
Cook Time: 6-8 mins / Total Time: 58 mins
Servings: 4 / Calories per serving:180 calories

Ingredients:
- 1 lb (450g) large shrimp, peeled and deveined
- 1/4 cup gluten-free soy sauce or tamari

- 2 tablespoons honey
- 2 cloves garlic, minced
- 1 tablespoon olive oil
- Wooden skewers, soaked in water

Method

Step 1

In a bowl, whisk together gluten-free soy sauce or tamari, honey, minced garlic, and olive oil to make the marinade.

Step 2

Thread the peeled and deveined shrimp onto soaked wooden skewers.

Step 3

Place the shrimp skewers in a shallow dish and pour the marinade over them. Make sure the shrimp are evenly coated. Let marinate in the refrigerator for at least 30 minutes.

Preheat the grill to medium-high heat. Remove the shrimp skewers from the marinade and discard any excess marinade.

Step 4

Grill the shrimp skewers for 3-4 minutes on each side, or until the shrimp are pink and cooked through.

Serve the grilled honey garlic shrimp skewers hot with your favorite side dishes.

Herb-Crusted Baked Cod:

Prep Time: 10 mins / Cook Time: 15-20 mins
Total Time: 30 mins / Servings: 4
Calories per serving: 220 calories

Ingredients:
- 4 cod filets
- 2 tablespoons olive oil
- 1 tablespoon Dijon mustard
- 1/4 cup gluten-free breadcrumbs
- 1 tablespoon chopped fresh parsley
- 1 teaspoon dried thyme
- Salt and pepper to taste

Method

Step 1
Preheat the oven to 400°F (200°C). Line a baking sheet with parchment paper.

Step 2
In a small bowl, combine olive oil and Dijon mustard. In another bowl, mix together gluten-free breadcrumbs, chopped fresh parsley, dried thyme, salt, and pepper.

Step 3
Brush the cod fillets with the olive oil and mustard mixture, then coat them evenly with the breadcrumb mixture.
Place the coated cod fillets on the prepared baking sheet. Bake in the preheated oven for 15-20 minutes, or until the fish is opaque and flakes easily with a fork.

Step 4

Serve the herb-crusted baked cod hot with lemon wedges and your choice of side dishes.

Turkey And Vegetable Stir-Fry:

Prep Time: 15 mins / Cook Time: 15 mins
Total Time: 30 mins / Servings: 4
Calories per serving: 280 calories

Ingredients:

- 1 lb (450g) turkey breast, thinly sliced
- 2 tablespoons gluten-free soy sauce or tamari
- 1 tablespoon sesame oil
- 2 cloves garlic, minced
- 1 teaspoon grated ginger
- 2 cups mixed vegetables (such as bell peppers, snow peas, carrots, and mushrooms)
- Cooked rice for serving

Method

Step 1

In a bowl, toss thinly sliced turkey breast with gluten-free soy sauce or tamari and grated ginger. Let marinate for 10-15 minutes.

Step 2

Heat sesame oil in a large skillet or wok over medium-high heat. Add minced garlic and stir-fry for 30 seconds, or until fragrant.
Add the marinated turkey breast to the skillet and stir-fry until cooked through.

Step 3

Add mixed vegetables to the skillet and stir-fry for 3-4 minutes, or until crisp-tender.
Serve the turkey and vegetable stir-fry hot with cooked rice.

Lemon Garlic Butter Scallops:

Prep Time: 10 mins / Cook Time: 5 mins
Total Time: 15 mins / Servings: 4
Calories per serving: 180 calories

Ingredients:

- 1 lb (450g) scallops, patted dry
- 2 tablespoons butter
- 2 cloves garlic, minced
- Zest and juice of 1 lemon
- Salt and pepper to taste
- Chopped fresh parsley for garnish

Method

Step 1
Pat dry the scallops with paper towels and season them with salt and pepper.

Step 2
Heat butter in a large skillet over medium-high heat. Add minced garlic and cook for 1 minute, or until fragrant.

Step 3

Add the scallops to the skillet in a single layer. Cook for 2-3 minutes on each side, or until they are golden brown and opaque in the center.

Add lemon zest and lemon juice to the skillet, stirring to coat the scallops evenly.

Serve the lemon garlic butter scallops hot, garnished with chopped fresh parsley.

GLUTEN-FREE DIPS, DRESSINGS, AND SAUCES

Guacamole

Prep Time: 10 mins /
Servings: 4
Calories per serving: 120 calories
Fat: 11g / Carbohydrates: 7g
Fiber: 5g / Protein: 2g

Ingredients:
- 2 ripe avocados
- 1 tomato, diced
- 1/4 cup finely chopped red onion
- 1/4 cup chopped fresh cilantro
- Juice of 1 lime
- Salt and pepper to taste

Method

Step 1.

Scoop the flesh of the avocados into a bowl and mash with a fork until smooth.

Step 2.
Stir in the diced tomato, chopped red onion, cilantro, and lime juice until well combined.

Step 3.
Season with salt and pepper to taste.

Step4.
Serve the guacamole with gluten-free tortilla chips or as a topping for tacos, salads, or grilled meats.

Homemade Salsa:

Prep Time: 10 mins / Chill Time: 30 mins
Servings: 6 / Calories per serving: 25 calories
Fat: 0.5g / Carbohydrates: 5g
Fiber: 1g / Protein: 1g

Ingredients:
- 3 ripe tomatoes, diced

- 1/2 red onion, finely chopped
- 1 jalapeño pepper, seeded and finely chopped
- 2 cloves garlic, minced
- Juice of 1 lime
- 1/4 cup chopped fresh cilantro
- Salt and pepper to taste

Method

Step 1.
In a bowl, combine diced tomatoes, chopped red onion, jalapeño pepper, minced garlic, lime juice, and chopped cilantro.

Step 2.
Season with salt and pepper to taste. Stir until well combined, then cover and refrigerate for at least 30 minutes to allow the flavors to meld.

Step 3
Serve the homemade salsa with gluten-free tortilla chips or as a topping for tacos, nachos, or grilled fish.

Honey Mustard Dressing:

Prep Time: 5 mins / Servings: 6
Calories per serving: 110 calories
Fat: 10g / Carbohydrates: 5g
Fiber: 0g / Protein: 0g

Ingredients:
- 1/4 cup Dijon mustard
- 2 tablespoons honey
- 2 tablespoons apple cider vinegar
- 1/4 cup olive oil
- Salt and pepper to taste

Method

Step 1.
In a small bowl, whisk together Dijon mustard, honey, and apple cider vinegar until smooth. Slowly drizzle in olive oil while whisking continuously until the dressing is emulsified.

Step 2

Season with salt and pepper to taste. Serve the honey mustard dressing over mixed greens or use it as a marinade for grilled chicken or vegetables.

Basil Pesto Sauce:

Prep Time: 10 mins / Servings: 6
Calories per serving: 200 calories
Fat: 20g / Carbohydrates: 2g
Fiber: 1g / Protein: 3g

Ingredients:

- 2 cups fresh basil leaves, packed
- 1/4 cup pine nuts
- 2 cloves garlic
- 1/2 cup grated Parmesan cheese
- 1/4 cup olive oil
- Salt and pepper to taste

Method

Step1.

In a food processor, combine fresh basil leaves, pine nuts, minced garlic, and grated Parmesan cheese. Pulse until the ingredients are finely chopped.With the food processor running, slowly drizzle in olive oil until the pesto reaches your desired consistency.

Step 2

Season with salt and pepper to taste. Serve the basil pesto sauce tossed with gluten-free pasta, spread on sandwiches, or as a dip for fresh vegetables.

Hummus:

Prep Time: 10 mins /
Servings: Makes about 2 cups
Calories per serving (2 tablespoons): 50 calories

Ingredients:

- 1 can (15 oz) chickpeas, drained and rinsed

- 2 cloves garlic, minced
- 1/4 cup tahini
- 2 tablespoons lemon juice
- 2 tablespoons olive oil
- 1/2 teaspoon ground cumin
- Salt to taste

Method:

Step1.
In a food processor, combine chickpeas, minced garlic, tahini, lemon juice, olive oil, ground cumin, and a pinch of salt.

2. Blend until smooth and creamy, scraping down the sides of the bowl as needed.

3. If the hummus is too thick, add a little water or additional olive oil to reach your desired consistency.

4. Taste and adjust seasoning with more salt or lemon juice if needed. Serve the hummus with

gluten-free crackers, raw vegetables, or as a spread on sandwiches and wraps.

Greek Yogurt Tzatziki Sauce:

Prep Time: 10 mins /
Servings: Makes about 1 cup
Calories per serving (2 tablespoons): 30 calories

Ingredients:
- 1 cup Greek yogurt
- 1/2 cucumber, grated and squeezed to remove excess moisture
- 2 cloves garlic, minced
- 1 tablespoon lemon juice
- 1 tablespoon chopped fresh dill
- Salt and pepper to taste

Method

1. In a bowl, combine Greek yogurt, grated cucumber, minced garlic, lemon juice, and chopped fresh dill.

2. Stir until well combined, then season with salt and pepper to taste.

3. Refrigerate for at least 30 minutes to allow the flavors to meld.

4. Serve the tzatziki sauce with grilled meats, falafel, or as a dip for pita bread and vegetables.

Creamy Avocado Lime Dressing:

Prep Time: 5 mins /
Servings: Makes about 1 cup
Calories per serving (2 tablespoons): 50 calories

- *Ingredients*:

1 ripe avocado, peeled and pitted
1/4 cup Greek yogurt
Juice of 2 limes
2 tablespoons chopped fresh cilantro
1 clove garlic, minced

2 tablespoons olive oil
Salt and pepper to taste

- Instructions:

1. In a blender or food processor, combine ripe avocado, Greek yogurt, lime juice, chopped cilantro, minced garlic, and olive oil.

2. Blend until smooth and creamy, adding water as needed to reach your desired consistency.

3. Season with salt and pepper to taste.

4. Serve the creamy avocado lime dressing over salads, grilled chicken, or as a dip for vegetable sticks.

Roasted Red Pepper Dip:

Prep Time: 5 mins /
Servings: Makes about 1 1/2 cups

Calories per serving (2 tablespoons): 40 calories

- **Ingredients**:

1 jar (12 oz) roasted red peppers, drained
1/2 cup Greek yogurt
2 tablespoons tahini
2 cloves garlic, minced
1 tablespoon lemon juice
1/2 teaspoon ground cumin
Salt and pepper to taste

- **Instructions**:

1. In a blender or food processor, combine roasted red peppers, Greek yogurt, tahini, minced garlic, lemon juice, ground cumin, salt, and pepper.

2. Blend until smooth and creamy, scraping down the sides of the bowl as needed.

3. Taste and adjust seasoning with more salt or lemon juice if needed.

4. Serve the roasted red pepper dip with gluten-free crackers, pita bread, or vegetable crudites.

Balsamic Vinaigrette Dressing:

Prep Time: 5 mins
Servings: Makes about 2/3 cup
Calories per serving (2 tablespoons): 80 calories

Ingredients:
1/4 cup balsamic vinegar
1/3 cup extra virgin olive oil
1 teaspoon Dijon mustard
1 clove garlic, minced
Salt and pepper to taste

Instructions:

1. In a small bowl, whisk together balsamic vinegar, extra virgin olive oil, Dijon mustard,

minced garlic, salt, and pepper until well combined.

2. Taste and adjust seasoning with more salt or pepper if needed.

3. Serve the balsamic vinaigrette dressing over mixed greens or use it as a marinade for grilled vegetables or meats.

Cilantro Lime Crema:

Prep Time: 5 mins / Servings: Makes about 1/2 cup
Calories per serving (2 tablespoons): 50 calories

Ingredients:
1/2 cup sour cream or Greek yogurt
Juice of 1 lime
2 tablespoons chopped fresh cilantro
1/2 teaspoon ground cumin
Salt and pepper to taste

Instructions:

1. In a bowl, whisk together sour cream or Greek yogurt, lime juice, chopped cilantro, ground cumin, salt, and pepper until smooth.

2. Taste and adjust seasoning with more salt or lime juice if needed.

3. Serve the cilantro lime crema as a topping for tacos, burritos, or grilled fish.

Chimichurri Sauce:

Prep Time: 10 mins / Servings: Makes about 1 cup
Calories per serving (2 tablespoons): 60 calories

Ingredients:
1 cup packed fresh parsley leaves
1/4 cup packed fresh cilantro leaves
2 cloves garlic, minced
2 tablespoons red wine vinegar
1/4 cup extra virgin olive oil

1/2 teaspoon red pepper flakes
Salt and pepper to taste

Instructions:

1. In a food processor, combine fresh parsley leaves, cilantro leaves, minced garlic, red wine vinegar, extra virgin olive oil, red pepper flakes, salt, and pepper.
2. Pulse until the ingredients are finely chopped and well combined.
3. Taste and adjust seasoning with more salt or red wine vinegar if needed.
4. Serve the chimichurri sauce drizzled over grilled steak, chicken, or vegetables.

Thai Peanut Sauce:

Prep Time: 5 mins / Servings: Makes about 1/2 cup
Calories per serving (2 tablespoons): 90 calories

Ingredients:

1/4 cup peanut butter

2 tablespoons gluten-free soy sauce or tamari

2 tablespoons lime juice

1 tablespoon honey

1 clove garlic, minced

1/2 teaspoon grated ginger

1/4 teaspoon red pepper flakes

Water as needed

Instructions:

1. In a bowl, whisk together peanut butter, gluten-free soy sauce or tamari, lime juice, honey, minced garlic, grated ginger, and red pepper flakes until smooth.

2. If the sauce is too thick, thin it out with water until you reach your desired consistency.

3. Taste and adjust seasoning with more soy sauce, lime juice, or honey if needed.

4. Serve the Thai peanut sauce as a dip for spring rolls, grilled chicken skewers, or drizzled over salads.

Sure! Here's a recipe for Spinach and Artichoke Dip with serving, prep, and cook information:

Spinach and Artichoke Dip

Servings: 6-8
Prep Time: 10 minutes
Cook Time: 20 minutes

Ingredients:
- 1 (10 oz) package frozen chopped spinach, thawed and drained
- 1 (14 oz) can artichoke hearts, drained and chopped
- 1 cup grated Parmesan cheese
- 1 cup shredded mozzarella cheese
- 1/2 cup mayonnaise
- 1/2 cup sour cream
- 1 teaspoon minced garlic
- 1/4 teaspoon salt
- 1/4 teaspoon black pepper
- 1/4 teaspoon red pepper flakes (optional)

- Tortilla chips, bread slices, or vegetable sticks for serving

Instructions:

1. Preheat your oven to 375°F (190°C).

2. In a mixing bowl, combine the drained spinach, chopped artichoke hearts, Parmesan cheese, mozzarella cheese, mayonnaise, sour cream, minced garlic, salt, black pepper, and red pepper flakes (if using). Mix until well combined.

3. Transfer the mixture into a baking dish and spread it out evenly.

4. Bake in the preheated oven for about 20 minutes, or until the dip is hot and bubbly, and the cheese is melted and golden brown on top.

5. Serve hot with tortilla chips, bread slices, or vegetable sticks for dipping.